MEDICAL ETHICS

MEDICAL SCHOOL CRASH COURSE

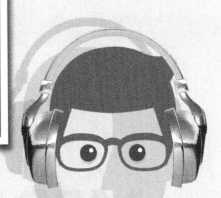

HIGH-YIELD CONTENT REVIEW

Q&A AND "KEY TAKEAWAYS"

TOP 100 TEST QUESTIONS

FOLLOW-ALONG PDF MANUAL

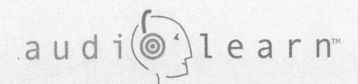

audiolearn™

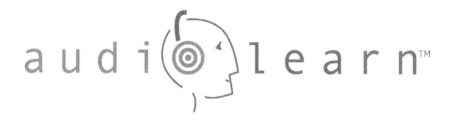

MEDICAL ETHICS

Medical School Crash Course™

www.AudioLearn.com

Table of Contents

Introduction: i

Chapter 1: Approaches to Ethics 1

The Four Principles of Medical Ethics 1

Approaches to Ethical Thinking 3

Utilitarianism & Consequentialism 3

Deontology Approach (Immanuel Kant) 5

Virtue Ethics (Aristotle) 6

Key Takeaways 7

Review Questions 8

Chapter 2: Patient Competence and Decision Making Capacity 12

Children and Adolescents 13

Mental Illness and Suicidal Patients 14

Altered Mental Status and Intoxicated Patients 15

Key Takeaways 16

Review Questions 17

Chapter 3: Confidentiality & Medical Records 21

Confidentiality 21

Exceptions to Confidentiality 22

Reportable Conditions 24

Medical Records and Digital Health 25

Key Takeaways 27

Review Questions 28

Chapter 4: Reproductive Health Ethics 33

Abortion 33

Historical Perspective 34

The Role of Feminism 35

Roe vs Wade 37

The Current State of Abortion in America 37

Maternal-Fetal Conflict 38

Role of Technology 38

Whose rights matter most? 39

The Question of Viability and Fetus' Rights 40

Accommodating Maternal Religious Beliefs 41

Sterilization 42

Types of Sterilization 43

Why do people choose sterilization? 43

Sterilization and Medical Ethics 44

Age and Patient Autonomy 44

Prejudice in Sterilization 45

The Murky Ethics of Physician Incentives 46

Unintended Consequences of Sterilization 47

Sterilization in the United States 47

Eugenics 47

Donation of Sperm and Eggs 49

Is this a rich person's problem? 50

Donor's Rights Versus Recipient's Rights 51

The Law on Egg Donation 52

Anonymity Versus Meeting the Donor 52

Sperm Donation 53

Donor's Rights in Sperm Donation 53

Key Takeaways 54

Review Questions 56

Chapter 5: End of Life Ethics **60**

Advance Directives 61

Withdrawal of Medical Treatment 62

Physician Assisted Suicide 63

Principle of Double Effect 64

Key Takeaways 65

Review Questions 66

Chapter 6: Physician Patient Relationship **71**

When does the relationship begin? 72

Confidentiality 73

Informed Consent and Shared Decision Making 74

Fiduciary relationship 76

Conflicts of Interest 78

Self-Care and Care for Family Members 78

Impaired Physicians 80

Relationships with Patients 80

Gifts from Patients 81

Medical Errors 82

Key Takeaways 82

Review Questions 84

Chapter 7: Ethics in Global Health **89**

Health as a Human Right 91

Social Determinants of Health 93

Organizations and Global Aid 94

Short term medical experiences 96

Brain Drain, Brain Gain, and Brain Circulation 98

Access to Medicines & The Role of Pharmaceutical Companies 100

Key Takeaways 102

Review Questions 103

Chapter 8: Research Ethics **108**

Informed Consent, Beneficence, and Non-maleficence 108

Nazi Experiments during World War II 109

1964 Declaration of Helsinki 111

Tuskegee Syphilis Experiments 111

HeLa Cells 112

Stem Cells 113

Key Takeaways 114

Review Questions 116

Chapter 9: Decision Making in Ethical Dilemmas **121**

Definition of an Ethical Dilemma 121

Non-maleficence - Do the benefits out-way any adverse risks to the patient? 122

Steps for Effective Decision-Making 122

Ethical framework for Decision-Making 123

"Rationing" of Limited Resources 124

START Triage 125

Conscientious Refusal 126

End of Life Care 127

Futile Care 129

Medical Ethics and the Law 130

Experimental Drugs and the Placebo.. 131

Hospital Ethics Committees.. 132

Key Takeaways.. 132

Review Questions 134

Summary: **139**

Review questions:.. **141**

Introduction:

The practice of medicine is a unique profession. One dedicated to service towards others in pursuit of healing, improved quality of life, and alleviation of suffering. Physicians are afforded a position of respect and power in society not just because of their proven intellectual ability, but also because of the ethical code they are expected to adhere to. This ethical code serves as the foundation upon which the doctor patient relationship is built.

Ethics can be defined as the framework to evaluate right versus wrong decisions according to an agreed upon set of underlying values. Medical ethics is the application of these principles to the field of clinical care and research. Medical ethics is considered distinct from medical law. While medical law is rigid and rule based, ethics requires flexible thinking based on circumstances, the patient's values or religious beliefs, and the provider's perspective. Guidance from medical ethics will therefore be both time and place specific, not absolute. Ethical guidance will depend on the norms and values of the local and on the norms and values of the specific providers and patients involved in the decision to be made.

Medical doctors have historically been held to a high standard of principles and values related to their decision making in clinical care, scientific research, and relationships with patients. The issue of medical ethics however, was brought into sharp focus during the Nuremberg trials of 1947 following the defeat of Nazi Germany in World War two. The trials revealed the participation of health professionals in the horrors of the Nazi regime. Their crimes included murder, torture, and medical experimentation without consent.

These trials led to a renewed interest in ethical standards for health providers. These standards are captured in the Hippocratic Oath- the pledge to adhere to ethical principles taken by physicians upon completion of their studies in many countries around the world. Hippocrates was a physician in ancient Greece and is often considered to be the father of the medical profession. His writings and teachings focused not only on the science and practice of medicine, but also on the philosophy of the physician patient relationship and the ethical responsibilities it entails. The original oath that bears his name dates back to the third century BC and has been updated several times to reflect the ages. The modern version most frequently used by medical school graduates was written in 1964 and reads as follows:

I swear to fulfill, to the best of my ability and judgment, this covenant:

I will respect the hard-won scientific gains of those physicians in whose steps I walk, and gladly share such knowledge as is mine with those who are to follow.

I will apply, for the benefit of the sick, all measures [that] are required, avoiding those twin traps of overtreatment and therapeutic nihilism.

I will remember that there is art to medicine as well as science, and that warmth, sympathy, and understanding may outweigh the surgeon's knife or the chemist's drug.

I will not be ashamed to say "I know not," nor will I fail to call in my colleagues when the skills of another are needed for a patient's recovery.

I will respect the privacy of my patients, for their problems are not disclosed to me that the world may know. Most especially must I tread with care in matters of life and death. If it is given me to save a life, all thanks. But it may also be within my power to take a life; this awesome responsibility must be faced with great humbleness and awareness of my own frailty. Above all, I must not play at God.

I will remember that I do not treat a fever chart, a cancerous growth, but a sick human being, whose illness may affect the person's family and economic stability. My responsibility includes these related problems, if I am to care adequately for the sick.

I will prevent disease whenever I can, for prevention is preferable to cure.

I will remember that I remain a member of society, with special obligations to all my fellow human beings, those sound of mind and body as well as the infirm.

If I do not violate this oath, may I enjoy life and art, respected while I live and remembered with affection thereafter. May I always act so as to preserve the finest traditions of my calling and may I long experience the joy of healing those who seek my help.

The Hippocratic Oath is infused with the core values of medical ethics, which include respect for patient autonomy, beneficence- or doing good for patients, non-maleficence- or not doing harm to patients, and justice. Ethical dilemmas arise when these values provide conflicting guidance with respect to specific scenarios confronting health practitioners. This course will present and discuss a variety of ethical dilemmas, along with a general overview to medical ethics. It will also provide an approach to ethical decision making in clinical situations and interpersonal interactions with patients and other health providers.

Chapter 1 provides an overview of medical ethics summarizing the core values of the field, which include respect for patient autonomy, beneficence - or doing good for patients, non-maleficence - or not doing harm to patients, and justice. The chapter then reviews three different philosophical approaches to ethical thinking including utilitarianism, deontology, and virtue ethics. These approaches stem from the philosophical teachings of Jeremy Bentham, John Stuart Mills, Immanuel Kant, and Aristotle, among others.

Chapter 2 discusses the issue of patient competence and decision making capacity, which is linked to the core value of respecting patient autonomy. This chapter discusses situations where patients may not have the ability to make decisions for themselves. The issues of informed consent, competence, and capacity will be reviewed here. The special cases of what to do when treating children, people with mental illness, or intoxicated patients will also be explored.

Chapter 3 highlights the importance of patient confidentiality and appropriate use of medical records, an issue that has become particularly important following the digital health revolutions of recent decades. This chapter will pay particular attention to exceptions to the confidentiality rule, including reportable conditions and moments where there is a concern for imminent harm.

Chapter 4 discusses one of the most controversial topics in medical ethics, covering issues related to reproductive health. The issue of abortion, for example, has become synonymous with medical ethics over recent decades. The issue becomes more complicated as technology related to fetal imaging and neonatal care continues to advance. Other topics included in this chapter are maternal fetal conflict, sterilization, and the donation of sperm and eggs.

Chapter 5 presents ethical dilemmas associated with end of life care, which have also grown more complicated alongside the advancement of medical science and technology. Physicians today have the ability to prolong human life as never before, but this begs the question: is it always beneficial to the patient to do so? Included in this chapter are discussions on advanced directives, withdrawal of treatment, medical futility, and physician assisted suicide.

Chapter 6 covers the physician patient relationship. The chapter defines when the relationship begins and highlights unique features of this relationship. These features include confidentiality, shared decision making, and the so called fiduciary relationship. It also discusses conflicts of interest, impaired physicians, inappropriate relationships between health providers and their patients, gifts from patients, and disclosure of medical errors.

Chapter 7 reviews ethical issues in global health. This chapter will cover dilemmas faced by Western health providers travelling to low resource settings to provide care. It will also discuss specific ethical issues around global health challenges such as health as a human right, the social determinants of health, ethics of the global fight against HIV/AIDS, and the issue of access to essential medicines in less developed countries.

Chapter 8 discusses ethics in medical research, including informed consent of human subjects and the ethics around new technologies including stem cells.

Chapter 9 concludes this course on medical ethics by providing a decision making framework to address ethical dilemmas. The utilization of review boards and ethics committees are discussed here as strategies to take action in the context of ethical conflict. Additional topics in the chapter include triage during mass casualties and rationing of scarce resources when the need for health services surpasses the health system's ability to provide it.

Chapter 1: Approaches to Ethics

The Four Principles of Medical Ethics

Physicians are confronted with ethical dilemmas, both small and large, every day that they practice their trade and care for patients. These dilemmas are often complicated by diverse opinions, points of view, religious convictions, and cultural perspectives. Practitioners, philosophers, and ethicists alike have struggled with these issues since the time of Hippocrates. Four guiding principles have emerged to define the boundaries of medical ethics and serve as a framework for thought.

These principles include respect for patient autonomy, beneficence - or doing good for patients, non-maleficence - or doing no harm to patients, and justice. These principles will be revisited in subsequent chapters as they relate to each specific topic of medical ethics. It is important to note here that no one value is weighed as greater than the other. The lack of hierarchy means that different providers or systems may come to different ethical conclusions or decisions when faced with a decision to be made.

The first principle is autonomy. Autonomy refers to a patient's individual right to consent to or refuse any course of treatment. They must be able to make these decisions free from coercion or threats. According to the principle of autonomy, the role of the physician is to inform the patient of the available treatment options and ultimately allow them to decide on their desired course of action. Unless a patient's mental state is impaired, for example by intoxication or psychiatric disease, patients should be empowered with the freedom to choose their own best course of action. Autonomy is the core value behind the concepts of informed consent and shared decision making related to medical treatment options. A patient's autonomy, or their personal decision to pursue or refuse treatment, can only be overruled in situations when their capacity is impaired. Examples of this impairment include intoxication, psychiatric illness, and dementia, or when a patient is unconscious and no designated decision maker is present.

The second principle is beneficence. The principle of beneficence states that physicians should only take actions that are beneficial for their patients by promoting well-being and improved health. They must therefore always strive to act in the best interests of their patients and to hold themselves to the highest moral standard. Beneficence in practice means weighing the benefits of any therapeutic action against its potential risks. It means protecting patients from harm or deterioration. It means taking actions aimed at improving the general welfare of patients, and keeping their best interests in mind rather than other considerations such as profit or other personal gains.

The beneficence principle is linked to the third principle, non-maleficence. Non maleficence states that physicians should not take any actions that cause harm to their patients. This principle is often summarized by the Latin phrase *primum non nocere*, or "first do no harm". Physicians must not take any action of malice or revenge against a patient. They should not administer an intervention that they know will cause the patient harm.

It is clear from the definitions as described that the principles of beneficence and non-maleficence are often in conflict. Physicians often attempt treatments they hope will be beneficial but may be associated with harmful side effects. An antibiotic might cure an infection, or it might cause an allergic reaction or induce a case of antibiotic associated diarrhea, for example. A course of chemotherapy might prolong a cancer patient's life by a few additional months, but the side effects of the therapy might be so severe that they enjoy a lower quality of life compared with undergoing no treatment at all.

The fourth principle is justice. Justice refers to a physician's respect for human rights and social justice with respect to their practice. This principle is concerned with human dignity, freedom, consent, equality, and fairness. Justice and human rights require that resources be distributed fairly. Human rights are usually reflected in the legal systems of countries, for example the United States Constitution, or by international treaties such as the Universal Declaration of Human Rights. To evaluate the justice principle of a decision, one must consider its legality and fairness. Actions that favor certain populations without justification, or that violate a person's individual rights, do not adhere to the principle of ethical justice.

Although the four principles appear straightforward and somewhat obvious, they are frequently in conflict with one another. Ethical dilemmas arise when one principle directs a physician towards a certain course of action, while another principle directs them to a different one. The field and study of medical ethics exists to address these dilemmas by providing frameworks of analysis and ethical thinking to utilize when approaching difficult decisions. Medical ethics institutions and committees provide a forum to discuss these dilemmas and also to help set an agreed upon protocol and precedent to assist when future issues arise.

Approaches to Ethical Thinking

Although there are a wide variety of approaches to ethical thinking, this chapter will focus on three commonly used frameworks. We will discuss utilitarianism, deontology, and virtue ethics.

Utilitarianism & Consequentialism

Utilitarianism, also known as consequentialism, evaluates decisions based on their outcomes, or consequences. This framework is often summarized by the phrase: "the ends justify the means." An ethical action or decision, utilizing this approach, would therefore be the one that does the most good or the least harm in a given situation. Put another way, an ethical action is one that produces a positive outcome, or at least the most positive outcome relative to other choices.

This approach was championed by Jeremy Bentham and John Stuart Mill in the eighteenth and nineteenth centuries. Benthem was an English philosopher who lived in the late 1700's and early 1800's. Along with his student and fellow philosopher John Stuart Mill, Bentham devised what he called the fundamental axiom of utilitarianism. According to his approach, and in his own words, this philosophy stated that "...it is the greatest happiness of the greatest number that is the measure of right and wrong." Benthem referred to this as the greatest happiness principle. He used his philosophical teachings to advocate for women's rights, the abolition of slavery, legal reform, and animal rights.

Taken to an extreme, utilitarian thinking means that doing harm to a few might be acceptable in certain circumstances if it eventually leads to a greater magnitude of good for the many. A classic example used to demonstrate utilitarian thinking was devised in the 1960's and is known as the runaway trolley thought experiment. The trolley problem has taken on a higher level of relevance in recent years with the development of autonomous vehicles with artificial intelligence. Algorithms featuring ethical decision making frameworks are now programmed into driverless vehicles to make similar decisions- should a computer driven car swerve to avoid a collision to save the passenger but endanger pedestrians, or should it do nothing and allow an accident to happen?

According to the trolley problem, a driver of a trolley or streetcar notices that the brakes have failed. Ahead of him on the track are five people who will be struck and killed if he does nothing. He has the ability to switch to an adjacent track, but that will mean killing a single person who is standing on track number two. So what action should the driver take? According to utilitarian thinking, the driver should switch tracks, killing the individual on the second track. Instead of killing five people, the trolley will have then only killed one, which is a better outcome in terms of maximizing benefit or minimizing loss. Of course, the analysis gets more complicated when additional factors are added in to the scenario. What if the one person on the adjacent track is a child and the five people on track one are elderly? What if the one person on track two is a loved one or relative? An important feature of this problem is that by switching tracks, the driver is altering the "natural" course of events and taking a direct action that alters another person's fate.

A common criticism of utilitarianism questions the so called observer who decides on the positivity or negativity of a consequence. Ideally, such an observer should be neutral and capable of identifying the full range of impacts resulting from an action. In practice however, this observer may be incapable of evaluating consequences beyond their limited scope of observation. An action may be judged as ethical by such a flawed observer despite having serious negative and unrecognized consequences.

Deontology Approach (Immanuel Kant)

Deontology or deontological ethics is an alternative ethical framework often contrasted with utilitarianism. This approach is often associated with eighteenth century German philosopher Immanuel Kant. Kant believed in what he called the categorical imperative, or unconditional rules that must be followed at all times in order to live a moral existence. For Kant, following these rules was important as an ends in and of themselves, not merely a means to improve a secondary outcome. In Kant's own words- "always recognize that human individuals are ends, and do not use them as a means to your end."

His theory of deontology relies on a belief in rules and moral duty related to an action rather than evaluating the outcomes of that action. An action can therefore be ethically right regardless of the outcome, as long as it is done with good intentions and according to universally agreed upon rules. Conversely, an action done with bad intentions and violating an agreed upon rule can never be considered ethical, even if it has a positive outcome. So deontology therefore supports universal moral rules. Do not steal. Do not cheat. Do not kill. Do not lie.

Revisiting the classic runaway trolley problem, deontology provides a different perspective. According to deontology, it would never be acceptable to take an action that would cause harm. So switching to track number two would be considered unethical since it would lead to a death. Here, the fact that the trolley driver takes an action that causes the death on track number two is important. It is differentiated from the driver taking no action and letting natural events take their course as the trolley collides with the five people on track number one.

This approach is in stark contrast to utilitarianism, which does not evaluate the action itself, only the outcome. Application of deontological thinking can often be problematic.

What if a criminal asks you for information that you know will allow them to do harm to someone. Do you lie, preventing the harm? Or do you tell the truth? Deontology requires you to tell the truth, since lying is wrong, but this means that you will knowingly facilitate harm done to another person. Strict deontological thinking is often criticized as it leads to outcomes that many would find unacceptable.

Virtue Ethics (Aristotle)

Finally, virtue ethics is a framework originating from Socrates, Aristotle, and several other philosophers of ancient Greece. This approach relies on an evaluation of moral character. Character here is defined as personal traits and core beliefs, which these philosophers referred to as virtues. Aristotle lists a variety of core positive virtues that must be developed through study, discipline, and self-awareness. These virtues include honesty, humility, generosity, and courage. Aristotle further differentiated the virtues into two categories, moral and intellectual. Moral virtues include temperance, fidelity, justice, and common sense. Intellectual virtues focus on knowledge and wisdom.

Each virtue listed, particularly the moral virtues, was considered a middle ground, or golden mean, between two extremes of character. Courage, for example, can be considered the middle ground virtue between recklessness on the one hand, and cowardice on the other.

Ethical decision making and analysis, according to virtue ethics, evaluates actions based on how they reflect an individual's character. It does not reflect on intentions or adherence to rules, which is the realm or deontology, nor does it evaluate the outcomes of the action as required by utilitarianism.

Ethical actions, according to virtue ethics, are those that would be taken by a virtuous person faced with similar circumstances. Virtuous people are individuals who make a conscious decision to live by the positive virtues previously discussed. So an ethical action in a dangerous situation would be one that a courageous person would take were they in the same situation.

Unfortunately for virtue ethicists, there is no agreed upon list of virtues to aspire to. The guidance it provides for ethical actions is also vague- how does a person truly know what a virtuous person would do if they are not virtuous themselves?

Key Takeaways

- The four principles of medical ethics are patient autonomy, beneficence, or doing good for patients, non-maleficence, or not doing harm to patients, and justice.

- Ethical dilemmas arise frequently and occur when any of the four principles conflict with each other.

- The discipline and practice of medical ethics aims to consider and resolve ethical dilemmas in healthcare. The outcome of many ethical dilemmas however, is decided by the legal system.

- Utilitarianism is an ethical theory that evaluates actions based on their consequences. The founders of this theory were Jeremy Bentham and John Stuart Mill. This framework is often summarized by the phrase: "the ends justify the means."

- Deontology is an ethical theory that evaluates actions based on their adherence to rules and responsibility. This theory is based on the writings and teachings of Immanuel Kant.

- Virtue ethics evaluates actions based on how they reflect an individual's character, or virtues. These virtues include honesty, humility, generosity, and courage. Ethical decision making and analysis, according to virtue ethics, evaluates actions based on how they reflect an individual's character. It does not reflect on intentions or adherence to rules, which is the realm of deontology, nor does it evaluate the outcomes of the action as required by utilitarianism.

1. Which of the following is a core principle of medical ethics?

    a. Freedom

    b. Autonomy

    c. Utilitarianism

    d. Courage

Answer: b. Autonomy refers to the patient's right to consent to and select their desired treatment. According to the principle of autonomy, the role of the physician is to educate the patient on the available treatment options and allow them to decide on their desired course of action.

2. What is the definition of non-maleficence?

    a. Do no harm

    b. Maximize benefit

    c. Promote well being

    d. Be honest

Answer: a. Non-maleficence states that physicians should not take any actions that cause harm to their patients. This principle is often summarized by the Latin phrase *primum non nocere*, or first do no harm.

3. Which of the following documents reflect the principle of justice in ethics?

    a. US Constitution

    b. Universal Declaration of Human Rights

    c. European Convention on Human Rights and Biomedicine

    d. All of the above

Answer: d. The principle of justice refers to physician respect for human rights and social justice with respect to their practice. This principle is concerned with human dignity, freedom, consent, equality, and fairness. Human rights are usually reflected in the legal systems of countries, for example the United States Constitution, or by international treaties like the Universal Declaration of Human Rights.

4. Which phrase summarizes the principle of utilitarianism?

    a. First do no harm

    b. Do unto others

    c. The ends justify the means

    d. To each according to their needs

Answer: c. Utilitarianism, also known as consequentialism, evaluates decisions based on their outcomes, or consequences. An ethical action or decision, utilizing this approach, would therefore be the one that does the most good or the least harm in a given situation. Put another way, an ethical action is one that produces a positive outcome.

5. Which philosopher is commonly associated with utilitarianism?

    a. Jeremy Bentham

    b. Aristotle

    c. Socrates

    d. Immanuel Kant

Answer: a. Jeremy Bentham is usually associated with utilitarianism. Benthem referred to his approach as the greatest happiness principle. Another philosopher associated with utilitarianism is John Stuart Mill.

6. Which philosopher is commonly associated with deontology?

    a. Jeremy Bentham

    b. Aristotle

    c. Socrates

    d. Immanuel Kant

Answer: d. Immanuel Kant is usually associated with deontology. Deontology relies on a belief in rules and moral duty related to an action rather than evaluating the outcomes of that action

7. Which philosopher is commonly associated with virtue ethics?

    a. Jeremy Bentham

b. Aristotle

c. Socrates

d. John Locke

Answer: c. Socrates and Plato are usually associated with virtue ethics. This approach relies on character traits and core beliefs, referred to as virtues. These virtues include honesty, humility, generosity, and courage.

8. Which of the following is an example of the golden mean in virtue ethics between recklessness and cowardice?

a. Honesty

b. Humility

c. Generosity

d. Courage

Answer: d. Each virtue described by virtue ethics is considered a middle ground, or golden mean, between two extremes of character. Courage, for example, can be considered the middle ground virtue between recklessness on the one hand, and cowardice on the other.

9. Which of the following ethical frameworks would characterize a particular action as wrong, even if it led to a positive outcome?

a. Virtue ethics

b. Utilitarianism

c. Deontology

d. All of the above

Answer: c. Deontology relies on a belief in rules and moral duty related to an action rather than evaluating the outcomes of that action. Any action that violates an agreed upon rule can never be considered ethical, even it has a positive outcome.

10. Which of the following ethical frameworks would justify telling a lie to avoid hurting someone's feelings?

a. Virtue ethics

b. Utilitarianism

   c. Deontology

   d. All of the above

Answer: b. Utilitarianism would value the care for the person's feelings over any rule against telling a lie. To the utilitarian the positive ends justify the negative means.

Chapter 2: Patient Competence and Decision Making Capacity

This chapter will review the issue of patient competence and decision making capacity. These topics are directly related to the core value of autonomy in medical ethics. Autonomy refers to the patient's ability and right to consent to and select their desired treatment. According to the principle of autonomy, the role of the physician is to educate the patient on the available treatment options and allow them to decide on their desired course of action. Autonomy is the core value behind the concepts of informed consent and shared decision making on medical treatment options. A patient must have the ability to safely and responsibly exercise their autonomy. This ability is known as competence.

Informed consent relies on a patient being of sound mind with intact decision making capacity. These patients are provided with the appropriate knowledge of treatment options, the consequences of each potential option, and costs and benefits of each approach. They must then be permitted to choose the option that best suits their values and desires, even if this choice contradicts the recommendation of a medical provider. An example of such a disagreement would be a case where a patient refuses a potentially lifesaving therapy, such as a blood transfusion, due to their religious beliefs. Decision making capacity evaluation is often summarized by the phrase- understanding, appreciation, reasoning, and ability to express a choice. These form a legal standard that relies on the patient's understanding of the care being offered, an appreciation of the consequences of compliance versus noncompliance, the ability to use reasoning to compare the various options, and the ability to express a discrete choice based on their analysis.

The issue of legal competence is separate from capacity, as it is a legal assessment of the patient's ability to make decisions. Under certain circumstances, a patient's autonomy can and must be overruled for their own good with a legal assessment of incompetence. This is done in order to protect their health and adhere to the value of beneficence-- doing good for the patient and acting in their best interest. These circumstances generally occur in the case of minors and in situations where patient capacity is impaired, including psychiatric illness, intoxication, and dementia.

Children and Adolescents

This section will discuss the issue of patient competency and decision making capacity as related to children and adolescents. As a general rule, a physician must obtain parental consent to treat any patient under the age of eighteen. The need for consent can be waived in the case of a life threatening or potentially life threatening condition. So, for example, epinephrine for a child presenting to the emergency room with an anaphylactic reaction should not be withheld while awaiting a call back from the child's parents. Conversely, a child with a stable medical complaint brought to the emergency room from school should not be treated until permission is obtained from their legal guardian.

Sometimes after permission to provide treatment is obtained from the legal guardian, children may not want to comply with the physical exam and may resist the treatments that are being provided to them. Although the cooperation of minors in their treatment is desirable, they are usually not considered to have the capacity to make medical decisions for themselves. In other words, they do not have the means to appreciate the consequences of their actions so are therefore unable to express a rational choice to refuse treatment. In cases where the minor patient disagrees with the decision of their parent or guardian, the guardian's decision takes precedent according the principle of beneficence.

In some states, minors may consent for themselves, without the need for an adult guardian, in certain situations. These usually include treatment of sexually transmitted diseases or for health care related to birth control or an active pregnancy. Some states even have a declared category for certain minors considered mature enough to make their own independent decisions. These so called "emancipated" minors are granted their status by a court order, by getting married, or by joining the military. An interesting nuance arises in the case of marriage, since minors require an adult guardian's permission to get married before the age of eighteen in the first place.

Emancipated minors are considered independent from parental control, and can therefore make healthcare decisions for themselves. Specific laws related to the ability of minors to consent for certain types of treatment and to become emancipated vary from state to state.

Mental Illness and Suicidal Patients

This section will discuss the issue of patient consent in cases of mental illness and suicidal patients. Nearly forty five thousand people commit suicide in the United States every year. Many of these people are in contact with health providers over the course of their mental illness, so health providers must make every effort to screen for and aggressively treat patients at risk for suicide. Severe mental illness is considered to be a condition where patients may not be competent to make their own decisions. Ethical standards support over ruling patient autonomy in cases where a patient is likely to harm others or themselves. This is once again done in the name of beneficence.

In most cases, even suicidal and mentally ill patients will cooperate with medical practitioners when brought to a healthcare setting. Treatments can then be administered with their consent. But what happens when a suicidal or mentally ill patient is brought to the emergency room by concerned family members or law enforcement officers, and they then refuse to cooperate and try to leave the facility? These patients must first be evaluated by a psychiatric professional in coordination with legal authorities before they can be permitted to leave the hospital. If they refuse to cooperate and attempt to leave during their evaluation, a temporary police detention order may need to be initiated to allow for the psychiatric evaluation to take place. This temporary order allows for patient to be placed in police custody while in the emergency room. They can then be evaluated by a psychiatrist and a decision can be made with the local magistrate as to how to proceed.

While specific laws vary from state to state, most agree that when patients are at imminent risk of self-harm or harm to others they can be transferred to a psychiatric facility against their will for a brief period of time. This process is known as involuntary, or civil, commitment.

Altered Mental Status and Intoxicated Patients

This section will discuss patient decision making capacity in intoxicated patients and patients with altered mental status. When patients demonstrate an acute alteration in their mental status associated with a medical illness or intoxication, they are not considered to be competent and able to refuse care. This conclusion is based on the assumption that, were they not confused from their illness or intoxication, they would consent to the treatments being offered.

In these situations, patients pose a danger to themselves and others. An intoxicated patient who refuses treatment at an emergency room and leaves the health facility can subsequently fall on the street or stumble into traffic. Even worse, they could attempt to drive themselves home and cause a serious accident, injuring innocent motorists and pedestrians.

Delirium and altered mental status can be the result of toxins like drugs or alcohol, systemic infections, cerebrovascular accidents, and head injuries, among other conditions. During the acute phase of treatment of these patients where there is an obvious medical cause, a psychiatric evaluation is usually not necessary. Physicians are expected to proceed with standard treatments including hospitalization, antibiotics, and intravenous fluids. Physicians should ensure that the medical record, that is- the patient's chart, reflects the patient's condition and the decision making process to administer treatments to an uncooperative patient.

If necessary, they may also be required to use chemical and physical restraints to prevent the patient from interfering with their treatment course. Chemical restraints, or sedative medications like lorazepam and haloperidol, are preferable to physical restraints.

- Informed consent relies on patients of sound mind with intact decision making capacity.

- Under certain circumstances, a patient's autonomy can and must be overruled for their own good in order to protect their health and adhere to the value of beneficence.

- A physician must obtain parental consent for any patient under the age of eighteen. This requirement can be waived in a case of a life threatening or potentially life threatening conditions.

- Although the cooperation of minors in their treatment is desirable, they are usually not considered to have the capacity to make medical decisions for themselves. This means that in cases where the minor patient disagrees with the decision of their parent or guardian, the guardian's decision takes precedent.

- Emancipated minors are considered independent from parental control, and can therefore make healthcare decisions for themselves. In some states, all minors may consent for themselves to the treatment of sexually transmitted diseases or for health care related to birth control or an active pregnancy. Emancipated minors are granted their status by a court order, by getting married, or by joining the military.

- Severe mental illness is considered to be a condition where patients may not be competent to make their own decisions. Ethical standards support over ruling patient autonomy in cases where a patient is likely to harm others or themselves.

- When patients demonstrate an acute alteration in their mental status associated with a medical illness or intoxication, they are not considered to be competent and able to refuse care. This conclusion is based on the assumption that, were they not confused from their illness or intoxication, they would consent to the treatments being offered.

1. Patient competence and decision making capacity is most associated with which core value of medical ethics?
    a. Autonomy
    b. Beneficence
    c. Non-maleficence
    d. Justice

Answer: a. Autonomy is the core value behind the concepts of informed consent and shared decision making on medical treatment options. Other core values include beneficence, or doing good, non-maleficence, or doing no harm, and justice.

2. Under which circumstance can a physician provide treatment to a minor without parental or legal guardian consent?
    a. Patient requests confidentiality
    b. Patient is a distant relative
    c. Patient has a life threatening injury
    d. All of the above

Answer: c. As a general rule, a physician must obtain parental or legal guardian consent for any patient under the age of eighteen. This need for consent can be waived in a case of a life threatening or potentially life threatening condition. If the patient is an emancipated minor then they can provide consent for their own care.

3. Which of the following is a common reason for a minor to be declared "emancipated"?
    a. Patient is married
    b. Patient is enlisted in the military
    c. Patient has a court order declaring them emancipated
    d. All of the above

Answer: d. "Emancipated" minors are granted their status by a court order, by getting married, or by joining the military. Emancipated minors are considered independent from parental control, and can therefore make healthcare decisions for themselves. Specific laws related to the ability of minors to consent for certain types of treatment and to emancipated minors vary state to state.

4. In a case of severe mental illness, under which scenario can a patient be transferred to a psychiatric facility against their will?
    a. Family member request
    b. Imminent threat to self
    c. Depression
    d. Disorganized thoughts

Answer: b. While specific laws vary from state to state, most concur that when patients are at imminent risk of self-harm or harm to others they can be transferred to a psychiatric facility against their will. This process is known as involuntary, or civil, commitment.

5. Under which of the following scenarios can a physician use chemical or physical restraints on an uncooperative patient?
    a. Intoxication
    b. Altered mental status from medical illness
    c. Delirium
    d. All of the above

Answer: d. When patients demonstrate an acute alteration in their mental status associated with a medical illness or intoxication, they are not considered to be competent. They are therefore unable to refuse care. This conclusion is based on the assumption that, were they not confused from their illness or intoxication, they would consent to the treatments being offered.

6. Which of the following statements is correct regarding chemical and physical restraints?
    a. Physical restraints are always preferable to chemical restraints
    b. When chemical restraints are used, the maximum dose should be administered

c. Physical and chemical restraints should be continued for the entire length of the patient's care regardless of the patient's condition

d. Chemical restraints at minimum effective doses are preferable to physical restraints

Answer: d. Chemical restraints, i.e. sedative medications, at minimum effective doses are preferable to physical restraints. Physical restraints like leather belts and vests can cause bruises or nerve injuries in patient and should only be used in cases where chemical restraints are not functioning or as a bridge to administering medications.

7. Which of the following is part of the definition of patient decision making capacity?
   a. Understanding
   b. Appreciation
   c. Reasoning
   d. All of the above

Answer: d. Decision making capacity evaluation is often summarized by the phrase: understanding, appreciation, reasoning, and ability to express a choice. These form a legal standard that relies on the patient's understanding of the care being offered, an appreciation of the consequences of compliance versus noncompliance, the ability to use reasoning to compare the various options, and the ability to express a discrete choice based on their analysis.

8. Which of the following statements about patient decision making are true?
   a. Capacity and legal competence are the same
   b. Capacity is determined by hospital administrators
   c. Legal competence is determined by the treating physician
   d. Legal competence is determined by legal authorities

Answer: d. Legal competence is determined by legal authorities. Physicians do not have the authority to declare a patient legally incompetent.

9. What steps are necessary when treating an uncooperative, suicidal patient?
   a. Medical evaluation

b. Psychiatric evaluation

c. Legal authority determination of competence

d. All of the above

Answer: d. Physicians cannot declare a patient legally incompetent. After a medical clearance, they must be evaluated by a psychiatric professional and then the case is referred to legal authorities. The patient may need to be placed in temporary police custody while these steps are in process.

10. Placing a patient into a psychiatric facility against their will is known as what type of commitment?

a. Voluntary commitment

b. Involuntary commitment

c. Judicial commitment

d. Medical commitment

Answer: b. While specific laws vary from state to state, most concur that when patients are at imminent risk of self-harm or harm to others they can be transferred to a psychiatric facility against their will. This process is known as involuntary, or civil, commitment. Voluntary commitment is when a patient checks themselves into a facility willingly.

Chapter 3: Confidentiality & Medical Records

Confidentiality

Confidentiality is specifically mentioned as a core principle to adhere to in the Hippocratic Oath. The phrase from the oath states: *I will respect the privacy of my patients, for their problems are not disclosed to me that the world may know.*

This chapter will discuss the issue of confidentiality related to physician patient interaction and medical records. Physicians have an ethical duty to keep patient information confidential. Medical records can only be shared with the patient's permission. This confidentiality can only be breached in the case of a few exceptions that will be discussed here.

Confidentiality aligns with a core value of medical ethics, justice. Justice here refers to the patient's right to be treated fairly in a safe and secure environment.

The issue of confidentiality also speaks to trust needed in the doctor patient relationship for medical care to be provided. Patients often must share private, intimate, potentially embarrassing personal details with their physician in order for the physician to provide adequate care. These issues can include sensitive issues related to reproductive health, sexual health, psychiatric disease, or substance abuse issues.

Without confidentiality, patients could fail to disclose critical details important to their diagnosis and treatment. Or they could refuse to seek treatment in the first place, worried about information related to their condition spreading to friends, family members, or law enforcement. A patient presenting to the emergency department with a complaint of chest pain, for example, may not feel comfortable disclosing their recent use of cocaine. This would lead the physician to consider treatment with anticoagulants for an acute coronary syndrome instead of providing benzodiazepines for cocaine induced coronary vasospasm.

Confidentiality in the doctor patient relationship is similar to that between an attorney and their client, often referred to as attorney client privilege. For physicians, the concept of physician patient privilege states that they should keep secret any information revealed during course of clinical care. In many legal jurisdictions, this privilege is recognized to the extent that physicians cannot be compelled to share patient information in court.

In practice, adhering to patient confidentiality standards requires vigilance against breaches in patient privacy. Physicians should adhere to the confidentiality guidelines to the best of their ability. Firstly, they should tell the patient when their information needs to be disclosed for clinical care purposes. This might include providing the patient's clinical information to other members of the provider care team or to consulting specialists. If a family member asks a question about their health situation, ask the patient first before sharing any details. Take care when discussing patient cases with colleagues in public places. Conversations in the hospital cafeteria or in building elevators where others may overhear details are inappropriate. Similarly, do not discuss patients on social media, and take special care to avoid mentioning details that could be used to identify a patient. Finally, when using patient cases for teaching purposes, remove all patient identifiers in order to mask their identity. In the United States, the law around patient identifiers is particularly strict following the Health Insurance Portability and Accountability Act of 1996, known as HIPAA, which will be described later in this chapter.

Exceptions to Confidentiality

This section will discuss exceptions to patient confidentiality. As a general rule, if maintaining patient confidentiality could theoretically cause an individual or group harm unless breached, then in that case disclosing the information may be allowable. The American Medical Association code on confidentiality concurs with this approach, allowing a breach of confidentiality only in the case of a threat of self-harm or harm to others or when there is a specific legal requirement to do so.

A common scenario already discussed in chapter two when a breach of confidentiality may be required occurs when a patient is mentally ill and either suicidal or homicidal. This threat of self-harm or harm to others may justify their involuntary commitment to a psychiatric hospital. It also justifies breach of their confidentiality in two specific ways. Firstly, if a patient reveals suicidal or homicidal thoughts during the course of a medical evaluation, the physician has a duty to report the situation to mental health professionals even if the patient requests that the physician keep their condition a secret. Secondly, a physician or psychiatrist evaluating a patient with a serious mental illness may need to contact their family members and disclose the patient's condition in order to solicit additional historical information.

Many legal jurisdictions around the world also require that health care practitioners notify law enforcement when they are treating a stab wound or gunshot wound. This notification must be made as soon as the condition is recognized and once the patient has been stabilized. The rationale for this reporting requirement is based on public safety. Reporting these types of injuries assists law enforcement with violent crime investigations and helps them protect the public from perpetrators of criminal acts. Some states even extend the principle to require mandatory reporting of all violent acts, not just those related to gunshot and stabbings.

Physicians and hospitals can be severely penalized for not reporting these cases when legally required to do so. In 2008, an NFL star athlete named Plaxico Burress accidentally shot himself with an unlicensed firearm. He contacted a local hospital in New York City before his arrival to seek care. The hospital then proceeded to knowingly provide him with treatment under an assumed name. The hospital and treating physician subsequently failed to notify law enforcement for nearly eight hours, and by that time the patient had already been discharged. As a result of this violation of the city's mandatory reporting law, the treating physician was suspended and an investigation was launched into the hospital's practices.

Cases of child abuse are another example where confidentiality must be breached. Medical decision making for children is, under normal circumstances, the responsibility of their adult legal guardians. In a circumstance where a medical provider suspects abuse, or when the child reports abuse to the provider, the provider is obligated to report the case to the police or other child welfare authority. These situations call into question the ability of legal guardians to provide a safe environment for the child. This scenario often arises when the injuries of a child do not match the history of the event provided by the child or family member. Specific concerning findings on physical examination may also arouse suspicion, including spiral bone fractures, retinal hemorrhages, and multiple old injuries at various stages of healing.

Finally, in many legal jurisdictions physicians must report impaired drivers to their local department of motor vehicles. This scenario could arise in the care of patient with a newly diagnosed seizure disorder, or for an elderly patient with worsening eyesight or dementia. These scenarios match the general approach to confidentiality exceptions since these drivers could put themselves and others at risk if they attempted to drive despite their medical conditions. It does however, put the treating physician in a difficult position as the act of reporting can have significant consequences for the patient in question. For many elderly patients, being able to drive themselves is important for them to maintain independence and to connect with social groups.

Reportable Conditions

This section discusses so called reportable conditions, which are another set of instances when patient confidentiality may need to be breached. Reportable conditions, also known as notifiable diseases, are diseases that a health provider must report to public health authorities when diagnosed. These conditions are determined and managed by local and national public health institutions like county and state health departments and the national Centers for Disease Control. Reports are submitted by physicians without the patient's permission and often include the patient's personal identifying information. Laws on reportable conditions force physicians to breach their patient's confidentiality. They must do so because the diseases included are considered to be important to public health and welfare. Reporting the diseases allows for public health officials to collect statistics, perform disease surveillance, and take direct interventions to ensure that outbreaks don't spread further. For example, the sexual contacts of a patient with a sexually transmitted disease may be notified, tested, and treated if necessary to prevent the disease from spreading onwards to their sexual partners in turn. This process is called contact tracing.

Some conditions require written notification to public health authorities, while others require immediate telephone notification. Others need only to be reported in aggregate, without patient data, or entered into registries. Examples of diseases requiring aggregate reporting include influenza and chickenpox. Cancer is a disease tracked by a registry.

Reportable conditions include highly contagious diseases, vaccine preventable diseases, and diseases that can be associated with bioterrorism. These diseases include measles, meningitis, rabies, anthrax, botulism, chlamydia, gonorrhea, syphilis, tetanus, and tuberculosis, to name a few.

In many states, partner notification laws exist related to HIV infected individuals. This means that if an individual is diagnosed with HIV, the physician has an obligation to inform their sexual partner or partners. The legal terminology for this obligation is known as the duty to warn. While it is not always possible for the physician to find and identify a patient's sexual partners, the law may state that they must make a good faith effort to do so. Health systems receiving money from the Ryan White HIV/AIDS program are required to adhere to this partner notification standard. The Ryan White program is an initiative funded by the federal government that supports HIV care for uninsured or underinsured individuals.

Medical Records and Digital Health

The proliferation of electronic medical records over the past decade has added a new dimension to the issue of patient confidentiality. It is now easier than ever to share or transmit patient data across digital platforms. The use of these electronic records can facilitate an individual patient's care, create opportunities for research, and promote public health.

In the pre-digital health record era, if a physician misplaced their briefcase they might expose up to a dozen patient files that they may have been carrying. In the digital era, a flash drive attached to a keychain can store a terabyte of data on many thousands of individuals. When networked and cloud based digital databases and platforms are breached, the private and confidential records of millions of patients can be compromised.

In the United States, rules regarding access to and sharing of such patient data were codified in the Health Insurance Portability and Accountability Act of 1996, commonly known as HIPAA. The law regulates the security of medical records and outlines circumstances under which records can be shared. The privacy rule of the Act specifically highlights the issue of protected health information, or PHI. PHI includes any information that can be used to link a medical record to an individual. While the medical record includes health conditions and treatments, patient identifiers under this framework include a patient's name, date of birth, social security number, medical record number, address, email, and photograph.

A medical record with PHI can only be shared or disclosed with a patient's written permission. Patients must also be granted access to their records and be able to request corrections if there are any inaccuracies. While these rules are in place to protect patient privacy, they sometimes create barriers to the provision of medical care. Imagine a semi-conscious patient arriving at the emergency room of a hospital where they have no recent records. In this situation, health providers may not be able to obtain written permission from the patient to obtain their records. Without written consent, they cannot call nearby hospitals to obtain the records, and this may hinder the patient's care.

- Confidentiality is specifically mentioned as a core principle to adhere to in the Hippocratic Oath. Confidentiality aligns with a core value of medical ethics, justice. Justice here refers to the patient's right to be treated fairly in a safe and secure environment.

- Without confidentiality, patients could fail to disclose details important to their diagnosis and treatment. Or they could refuse to seek treatment in the first place, worried about information related to their condition spreading to friends, family members, or law enforcement.

- As a general rule, if maintaining patient confidentiality could cause an individual or group harm, then in that case disclosing the information may be allowable. The American Medical Association code on confidentiality concurs with this approach, allowing a breach of confidentiality only in the case of a threat of self-harm or harm to others or when there is a legal requirement to do so.

- Many legal jurisdictions around the world also require that health care practitioners notify law enforcement when they are treating a stab wound or gunshot wound. The rationale for this reporting requirement is based on public safety.

- In a circumstance where a medical provider suspects child abuse, or when a child reports abuse to the provider, the provider is obligated to report the case to the police or other child welfare authority even if the child or their adult guardian requests confidentiality.

- In many legal jurisdictions physicians must report impaired drivers to their local department of motor vehicles.

- Reportable conditions, also known as notifiable diseases, are diseases that a health provider must report to public health authorities when diagnosed. Reporting the diseases allows for public health officials to collect statistics, perform disease surveillance, and take interventions to ensure that outbreaks don't spread further.

- In the United States, rules regarding access to and sharing of patient data were codified in the Health Insurance Portability and Accountability Act of 1996, commonly known as HIPAA. The law regulates the security of medical records and outlines circumstances under which records can be shared

Review Questions

1. Which core value of medical ethics does patient confidentiality most closely align?
    a. Autonomy
    b. Beneficence
    c. Non Maleficence
    d. Justice

Answer: d. Confidentiality aligns with a core value of medical ethics, justice. Justice here refers to the patient's right to be treated fairly in a safe and secure environment. Beneficence refers to physicians attempting to do good. Non maleficence means that they should strive to do no harm.

2. Which of the following is a reason that patient confidentiality is important to medical care?
    a. Allows patients to share private information to help their physician make the right diagnosis
    b. Prevents law enforcement from accessing medical records when crimes are committed
    c. Prevents insurance companies from accessing medical records to bill patients
    d. All of the above

Answer: a. Patients often must share private, intimate, potentially embarrassing personal details with their physician in order for the physician to provide adequate care. These issues can include sensitive reproductive, sexual health, psychiatric, or substance abuse issues. Without confidentiality, patients could fail to disclose details important to their diagnosis and treatment. Or they could refuse to seek treatment in the first place, worried about information related to their condition spreading to friends, family members, or law enforcement.

3. Which of the following cases represents a breach in patient confidentiality?
   a. Transmitting medical records to another physician with written permission from the patient
   b. Discussing the patient's medical condition with a consulting physician
   c. Disclosing an adult patient's diagnosis to their family member who asks for an update
   d. All of the Above

Answer: c. In practice, adhering to patient confidentiality standards requires vigilance against breaches in patient privacy. Physicians should tell the patient when their information needs to be disclosed for clinical care purposes. If a family member asks a question about their health situation, ask the patient first before sharing any details. Discussing medical details with a consulting physician treating the same patient is not a breach of confidentiality. Records can be transmitted to other parties if a patient provides written permission to do so.

4. Which of the following is a potential scenario when patient confidentiality may be breached (depending on the legal jurisdiction)?
   a. Gunshot wound report to the police
   b. Stab wound report to the police
   c. Impaired driver report to the department of motor vehicles
   d. All of the above

Answer: d. As a general rule, if maintaining patient confidentiality could cause an individual or group harm, then in that case disclosing the information may be allowable. The American Medical Association code on confidentiality concurs with this approach, allowing a breach of confidentiality only in the case of a threat of self-harm or harm to others or when there is a legal requirement to do so. Gunshot and stab wounds are often required to be reported to the police in the interest of public safety and to aid in criminal investigations. Impaired drivers must be reported in order to prevent them from driving and causing accidents.

5. Which of the following scenarios are suspicious for child abuse and should be reported to child welfare authorities?
    a. Sprained ankle in 11 year old while playing soccer
    b. Spiral forearm fracture in 2 year old who fell from bed
    c. Finger crush injury in 8 year old whose hand was caught in the car door
    d. All of the above

Answer: b. Cases of child abuse are another example where confidentiality must be breached. In a circumstance where a medical provider suspects abuse, or when the child reports abuse to the provider, the provider is obligated to report the case to the police or other child welfare authority. This scenario often arises when the injuries of a child do not match the history of the event provided by the child or family member. Concerning findings on physical examination may also arouse suspicion, including spiral bone fractures, retinal hemorrhages, and multiple old injuries at various stages of healing.

6. What is the benefit of breaching confidentiality in the case of reportable conditions or notifiable diseases?
    a. Allows public health officials to collect disease statistics
    b. Disease surveillance
    c. Allows public health officials to prevent diseases from spreading further
    d. All of the above

Answer: d. All of the above. Laws on reportable conditions force a physician to breach their patient's confidentiality. Reportable conditions, also known as notifiable diseases, are diseases that a health provider must report to public health authorities when diagnosed. These conditions are determined and managed by local and national public health institutions like county and state health departments and the national Centers for Disease Control. Reports are submitted by physicians without the patient's permission and often include the patient's personal identifying information. Laws on reportable conditions force physicians to breach their patient's confidentiality. They must do so because the diseases included are considered to be important to public health and welfare. Reporting the diseases allows for public health officials to collect statistics, perform disease surveillance, and take direct interventions to ensure that outbreaks don't spread further. For example, the sexual contacts of a patient with a sexually transmitted disease may be notified, tested, and treated if necessary to prevent the disease from spreading onwards to their sexual partners in turn. This process is called contact tracing.

7. Which of the following diseases is a reportable or notifiable disease?
   a. Syphilis
   b. Pneumonia
   c. Respiratory Syncytial Virus
   d. Coronavirus

Answer: a. Reportable conditions include highly contagious diseases, vaccine preventable diseases, and diseases that can be associated with bioterrorism. These include measles, meningitis, rabies, anthrax, botulism, chlamydia, gonorrhea, syphilis, tetanus and tuberculosis, to name a few. Some conditions require written notification to public health authorities, while others require immediate telephone notification. Others need only to be reported in aggregate, without patient data, or entered into registries. Examples of diseases requiring aggregate reporting include influenza and chickenpox. Cancer is a disease tracked by a registry. Reportable conditions include highly contagious diseases, vaccine preventable diseases, and diseases that can be associated with bioterrorism.

8. Which of the following are a common category of a notifiable condition?
   a. Highly contagious diseases
   b. Vaccine preventable illnesses
   c. Diseases associated with bioterrorism
   d. All of the above

Answer: d. Reportable conditions include highly contagious diseases, vaccine preventable diseases, and diseases that can be associated with bioterrorism. These include measles, meningitis, rabies, anthrax, botulism, chlamydia, gonorrhea, syphilis, tetanus and tuberculosis, to name a few.

9. Which US law regulates the access and sharing of patient data, including digital data?
    a. Patient Protection and Affordable Care Act
    b. Record Privacy Act
    c. Health Insurance Portability and Accountability Act
    d. Smoot-Hawley tariff Act

Answer: c. In the United States, rules regarding access to and sharing of such patient data were codified in the Health Insurance Portability and Accountability Act of 1996, commonly known as HIPAA. The law regulates the security of medical records and outlines circumstances under which records can be shared. A medical record with personal health information (PHI) can only be shared or disclosed with a patient's written permission. Patients must also be granted access to their records and be able to request corrections if there are any inaccuracies. While these rules are in place to protect patient privacy, they sometimes create barriers to the provision of medical care.

10. Which of the following is considered protected health information or PHI?
    a. Laboratory Results
    b. Digital x-ray images
    c. Diagnosis billing code
    d. Medical record number

Answer: d. PHI includes any information that can be used to link a medical record to an individual. While the medical record includes health conditions and treatments, patient identifiers under this framework include a patient's name, date of birth, social security number, medical record number, address, email, and photograph.

Chapter 4: Reproductive Health Ethics

This section will discuss one of the most controversial topics in medical ethics- reproductive health ethics. Reproductive health ethics is an important topic because of both social changes and advancements in technology. Women are choosing to have children at a later age, and what families look like has evolved- no longer must there necessarily be a male and a female as the parental unit – though this remains the norm. Families can consist of two mothers, two fathers, or single parents who have achieved their reproductive goals either through natural methods or with the assistance from modern technology.

Changes in reproductive technology have brought about exciting new methods available for those interested in being parents, to whom being pregnant or having a biological child would have been impossible in the past. These new technologies bring with them new challenges. This chapter will attempt to explore topics such as: abortion and the Supreme Court case Roe versus Wade, maternal-fetal conflict, sterilization, and the donation of sperm and eggs.

Abortion

We will first address the contentious medical ethics around abortion. Abortion means, essentially, electively terminating a pregnancy. Around the world it is one of the most controversial topics in medical ethics– and it has been a hot button issue in the United States for quite some time. Those who are against abortion fall into the "pro-life" camp, whereas those who are for women having the right to choose are called, appropriately, "pro-choice." Opinions and legal contexts differ as to if the procedure should be legal, the timeframe during the pregnancy when it is allowable, and under what conditions it can be performed. Some people, for example, believe that abortion should only be allowed in cases of rape or when the pregnancy poses a danger to the health of the mother.

From the perspective of medical ethics, it's clear to see why abortion is such a controversial topic for physicians. Being pro-choice means that doctors prioritize a woman's right to govern her own body, which falls under respect for patient autonomy. They may have to separate their own views on the topic from the wishes of the patient. Helping a woman have an abortion because she chooses to do so may also fall under the principle of beneficence, which means doing good for patients. A woman would be more empowered and perhaps be happier because she was able to make a choice for herself. In the case of pregnancy that could be dangerous or even fatal for a mother, doctors would be performing a life-saving procedure.

Saving a mother's life is clearly a case of beneficence when looking from the perspective of her physician, but there are multiple viewpoints on abortion. It's when one examines the issue from the perspective of the fetus that medical ethics can become unclear. Performing an abortion requires the termination of the life of a fetus. Being pro-life hinges on the principle of non-maleficence, or not doing harm to patients, if one looks at the issue from the perspective of the fetus. Controversy arises from when one believes that life begins. Those who believe that life begins at conception clearly are at a conundrum when looking at a mother's health versus that of her fetus, and have to balance the idea of beneficence of the mother with that of non-maleficence towards the fetus.

Historical Perspective

It may be surprising to know that abortion was not always such a divisive issue. According to Leslie Reagan, a professor of history at the University of Illinois, Urbana-Champagne, it was actually once a booming business in America. From 1800 till about 1880, it was legal and easy to buy drugs to induce abortion, as well as to get access to doctors to perform invasive procedures to carry it out. So, what changed?

According to Professor Reagan's book, "When Abortion Was a Crime," the practice became illegal in 1880 not due to morality, but to issues of health and safety. Concerns were raised related to poisoning caused by the drugs used to induce abortion. It was in fact doctors who pushed for abortion to become illegal. This fell under the principle of non-maleficence: doctors were concerned that circulating medications were causing harm to patients. Incidentally, it was only in 1869 that abortion was condemned by the church.

The American Medical Association, or AMA, which today fights for the rights of doctors to best treat their patients without government interference, began lobbying the government to make abortion illegal back in 1857. Reagan argues that some of the lobbying efforts were not solely from a medical perspective, but also from an anti-feminist one. One of the most prominent anti-abortion crusaders was Dr. Horatio Storer. He was a graduate of Harvard Medical School. And the timing of his actions was quite interesting: it coincided with a burgeoning movement of women pushing to be allowed to study at Harvard Medical School.

There was also pressure from legislators to criminalize abortion, particularly from one Anthony Comstock. His efforts paid off, and in 1873, the United States Congress passed the Comstock Law. This law was more concerned with moral aspects as opposed to patient health. The Comstock Law made it illegal to produce, publish and distribute material on how to get an abortion, among other things. Comstock's moral crusade, combined with doctors' own medically motivated concerns about unsafe abortions, led to the practice being made a felony crime in all states by 1900.

While the criminalization of abortion was universal in America, some states outlined exceptional circumstances that allowed for the practice to be performed. These circumstances included pregnancy as a result of rape or incest and also when the mother's life was in danger. In this latter case, it was agreed in these locations that the ideal of beneficence to the mother outweighed the non-maleficence to the fetus.

The Role of Feminism

Despite abortions being illegal, they continued to be performed, largely through networks of clandestine health providers. Women's groups increasingly pushed for the right to choose in order to control their reproductive destinies, and this quickly grew into a movement. One notable person in the movement was an activist named Margaret Sanger. In 1921, she founded the American Birth Control League or ABCL, an organization dedicated to pushing for the creation and promotion of birth control clinics. Sanger believed that women had the right to control their own fertility, and this included access to abortion. In 1942, the ABCL went on to become an organization that is likely familiar to listeners: the Planned Parenthood Federation of America. Due to the actions of ABCL and other pro-choice groups, abortions continued to be offered to many, though not all, women who requested them despite the practice being illegal.

Many physicians had similar views to those espoused by the American Birth Control League and performed pregnancy termination procedures in their clinics. It is estimated that they were performing 800,000 abortions a year by 1930. Many women who didn't have access to legal abortions or clandestine abortions in a physician's office however, were forced to undergo dangerous illegal ones. These were often conducted by unscrupulous characters in unsanitary conditions and could result in extreme illness or death.

One woman who played a reluctant role in this movement was Sherri Finkbine, who learned that the baby she was carrying – her fifth child – was likely to have severe limb deformities as a result of a medication she was taking during her pregnancy, Thalidomide. Finkbine spoke out about the issue because she wanted to warn other women about the dangers of the drug, which was popular at the time. She also wanted an abortion, but the state she lived in, Arizona, only allowed the procedure if the mother's life was at risk. Unwilling to put her life at risk by seeking out an illegal abortion, she instead flew to Sweden in 1962 to have the procedure.

Like Sherri Finkbine, Gerri Santoro also became a key figure in the pro-choice movement: she died due to complications from an illegal abortion in 1964. This galvanized women to train to perform safe abortions themselves, even though they were still illegal at the time. To them, this was an example of the ethical principle of beneficence: the need to provide a safe procedure for the well-being of a patient as opposed to sending them to dangerous underground providers, where the safety of the procedures available was uncertain. It also fell under the scope of patient autonomy: allowing a patient, in this case, a woman, to make decisions about her own body herself.

Roe vs Wade

Roe vs Wade was a legal ruling that remains synonymous with the battle for women's right to abortion in the United States. The landmark decision by the United States Supreme Court in 1973 ruled in favor of a woman's right to an abortion. In their decision, Supreme Court justices cited the fourteenth amendment of the Constitution, which cited a woman's right to privacy.

Again, it was a woman who fought for this right, a Texan named Norma McCorvey, who was referred to in court documents as Jane Roe. McCorvey was pregnant with her third child in 1969. She decided to go against the advice of her friends to lie and claim that she was raped in order to argue for an abortion in Texas. At the time, Texas law only allowed abortion when the mother's life was in danger, but may have also allowed the procedure in cases of rape. McCorvey wanted to fight for her rights and went to court, where she battled against Henry Wade, who was the District Attorney of Dallas County at the time. Sarah Weddington and Linda Coffee served as her legal representation. The case worked its way through the legal system over the following three years before receiving a verdict in her favor at the Supreme Court level. In the meantime, she gave birth to a child who was later adopted.

Before Roe vs Wade, access to abortions was restricted in most states. Thirty states did not allow for abortions for any reason at all, whereas 16 states allowed for abortions in specific circumstances, varying from rape, incest, and danger to the mother's life. Roe vs Wade allowed for access to abortion within the first trimester or twelve weeks of a fetus' existence. After this period, the court said a woman could still have access to abortion if the mother's life or health was in any danger.

The Current State of Abortion in America

Despite the Roe vs Wade Supreme Court ruling in 1973, the abortion debate has not disappeared and is alive and well in politics today. The longevity of the debate is simple- there is no clear-cut answer as to when life begins. While abortion remains legal, many states have sought to curtail it through statewide legislation. Legislation can restrict abortion by raising the bar on physician licensing to perform the procedure, clinical capacity of the clinic where the procedure is performed, and requiring counseling and waiting periods for the pregnant woman before she can access the procedure. Iowa, Mississippi, and Texas are among the states that currently have highly restrictive laws on the books related to abortion.

Maternal-Fetal Conflict

We will now move on to a topic related to abortion but not limited to it- maternal-fetal conflict. Maternal fetal conflict occurs when the health or interests of the mother are in conflict with the needs of the growing fetus.

A gynecologist or obstetrician dealing with pregnancy is in a unique position compared to other doctors: he or she is looking out for the interest of not one life, but two. The physician must think of the needs of both the mother and the unborn child, making medical ethics particularly fraught at this time. What happens when the mother does not comply with treatments or uses dangerous illegal substances? How does the physician act in the best interest of the fetus? Conversely, what happens when a mother is willing to put her own health at risk to better serve the interest of her unborn child in the case of pregnancy complication?

Role of Technology

According to Dr. Mary Jo Ludwig, a professor of medicine at the University of Washington, issues of medical ethics related to maternal-fetal conflict are on the rise. Dr. Ludwig argues that this is the case due to advances in technology. Improved technology means that physicians are better able to detect potential problems at earlier stages of a pregnancy. It also means that they can be more interventionist, which means they are able to do more procedures on the fetus than in previous eras.

These advances in technology have changed the way physicians look at pregnant women: previously, they viewed a mom and baby as, what Dr. Ludwig calls, "one complex patient." They looked at medical interventions under this lens. The medical model on pregnancy has moved from one focused on "unity to duality," according to Dr. Ludwig. Doctors now look at what is best for the mother and the fetus, treating them as separate patients.

Whose rights matter most?

Challenging situations can arise when helping a fetus could hurt the health of the mother, or the other way around. In terms of medical ethics, this would be a case of beneficence for one party as opposed to non-maleficence to the other. Pregnancy, even in the best circumstances, comes with some risks to the mother. The fetus is, after all, taking energy from her body to grow. But what happens when a physician must make a decision that favors the health of one over the other?

This isn't a case of choosing between two separate patients because the patients are linked. It would be much like choosing what to do with a set of conjoined twins, who are separate yet together. Most mothers care about their children and will do their utmost to ensure their children are in good health, sometimes putting themselves under great risk. This was the case for Danielle Dick, of Kansas. Dick was diagnosed with stage four melanoma in April 2017. She was seventeen weeks pregnant and she was carrying twins. Dick made the decision to delay radiation treatment as it could kill the fetuses she was carrying. Her children were born at twenty nine weeks in July 2017. Danielle Dick paid the ultimate sacrifice as a result of her decision to delay her own care: she died in April 2018.

Not all parents are as self-sacrificing as Danielle Dick. Some may suffer from conditions where they would not be able to function without treatment, though the treatment itself may be harmful to their fetus. One example of this would be pregnant women who are addicted to opioids and taking methadone in order to have supervised withdrawal from their addiction. Babies born to those taking opioids or methadone can be addicted to the substances upon birth. After birth, they begin to exhibit symptoms of drug withdrawal which can be life threatening. This condition is called neonatal abstinence syndrome or NAS.

Some doctors encourage pregnant women to give up their opioids without the help of methadone, the cold turkey approach, with the hope that the fetuses will not develop NAS.

Other physicians recognize the seriousness of this addiction and the challenge that these mothers face. It is not simply a case of willpower and determination in terms of the chemical addictions. It is here where one has to make the careful decision on what to advise: something that works for the benefit of the mother, highlighting the principle of beneficence, or something that will not harm the fetus, falling under the ethical principle of non-maleficence. If a doctor forces a mother to withdraw from a drug unassisted, she may relapse and overdose, in which case, both mother and fetus would be harmed.

The Question of Viability and Fetus' Rights

When deciding whether or not a mother's rights trump those of a fetus, similar ethical issues arise in the case of abortion. This arises primarily because there is still a great deal of debate as to the point in time at which a fetus becomes a person and has rights of their own. The University of Washington's Dr. Ludwig points out that in most of the world, pregnant women's rights take precedence over the rights of their fetuses. As in the case of abortion, a fetus' rights increase as it gets older. As a reminder, abortion is legal in the United States in the first trimester and part of the second trimester depending on the state.

Some ethicists say that the rights of a fetus are tied to viability. Viability means being physically able to live outside of the mother's body. The older the fetus is, the more viable it is, culminating at birth, when it is a separate human being from its mother.

Other medical ethicists say that treating fetuses like people means that their mothers are simply treated as carriers and their wishes are not important. On the other hand, this does not mean that a fetus has no rights at all. Pregnant women are legally obligated – up to a certain level – to not harm their fetus. They can even be charged with fetal abuse if they refuse hospitalization or intrauterine transfusions when medically necessary. In these cases, it is once again two principles of medical ethics battling each other: a woman's right to patient autonomy versus non-maleficence of the fetus.

What happens when medical intervention is required for the health of the fetus but the mother refuses it due to religious or cultural grounds? According to an article in the American Medical Association's Journal of Ethics in May 2005, adults can refuse treatment on religious grounds. They have the freedom, or autonomy, to choose. The article's author, Faith Lagay, says that the case is not so clear cut when a woman is making a decision that could engender the health of her unborn child.

One example of such a situation is known as *In re Fetus Brown*. Darlene Brown, a thirty four year old pregnant woman, went to the hospital for urinary discomfort only to discover that she needed surgery to remove a urethral mass. During the surgery, Brown lost a lot of blood and her hemoglobin levels dropped to one third of what they should be for a woman at that stage of her pregnancy. Her physician, Dr. Robert Walsh, requested a blood transfusion, but was informed by Brown – who was awake during the procedure – that she was a Jehovah's Witness. Jehovah's Witnesses do not believe in receiving blood transfusions as part of their religious beliefs. Dr. Walsh was able to complete the surgery without a transfusion, but asked for court approval as, according to Lagay, he believed that transfusions would be life-saving for both Brown and her fetus.

The Illinois circuit court subsequently held a hearing during which they named a hospital administrator as the temporary custodian of Fetus Brown. The hospital administrator decided in favor of blood transfusions to be administered in order to save the fetus' life, and over the next day-and-a-half, multiple transfusions were given to Darlene Brown against her will. She continued to be vehemently against these transfusions as they interfered with her religious beliefs – so much so that she had to be restrained and sedated in order to get them. Fetus Brown became baby Brown three days later – he was born healthy thanks to these transfusions, and the court removed the hospital administrator's custodianship a week later.

Despite her life and that of her baby being saved by the transfusions, Brown was very upset at having her religious beliefs ignored. She filed a court appeal because she believed that she was entitled to make medical decisions for herself, which falls under the principle of patient autonomy in medical ethics. The court ruled that this case was moot as the custodianship was lifted at the time of Brown's appeal and Fetus Brown was now an autonomous individual. But it nevertheless decided to consider the case as it was important for precedence in future cases.

The circuit court argued in favor of its decision for two reasons: first, it did not think that a blood transfusion was an invasive procedure, and, second, the court looked at the interest of the state versus the mother, as opposed to the fetus versus the mother's interests. The issue of viability played into the state's decision to act as it did. As you recall, viability is an issue in deciding how developed a fetus can be before an abortion is allowed.

In the end, the appeals court ruled in favor of Darlene Brown and against the circuit court. It said that a blood transfusion was indeed considered to be an invasive procedure. It also ruled that a woman's right to patient autonomy applied even if she was pregnant.

In re Fetus Brown has clear implications on the legality on medical treatment for pregnant women today. State laws do not allow pregnant women to be forced to undergo a medical treatment if they refuse due to religious reasons. They say that not one but two ethical rules are being broken by doing so: a woman's right to patient autonomy as well as her human right to practice a religion.

Legalities aside, the topic of maternal-fetal conflict is one fraught with tension and can be challenging for physicians as time is often of the essence and running to courts may not be an option. This is a reason why legal precedence and ethical guidelines are so important related to this topic.

Sterilization

We are now going to discuss the issue of sterilization. Sterilization refers to a number of medical techniques, many of which differ depending on the sex of the patient, that leave an individual unable to biologically reproduce. In the literal sense, sterilization is a form of birth control. Sterilization procedures vary and also have two important differences: some are permanent, while others are reversible. Most methods are considered permanent and reversing them, while sometimes theoretically possible, tend to be exceedingly difficult. Sterilization – when adding female and male numbers together – is the most common form of birth control in the United States.

Types of Sterilization

There are several different methods of sterilization. Two of the most popular kinds of sterilization are vasectomies and a tubal sterilization. A vasectomy is a surgical procedure for men. It consists of cutting the vas deferens – which are the tubes that carry sperm from the testicles to the prostate. This prevents the sperm from entering semen, hence rendering a man unable to reproduce since their ejaculate will be devoid of sperm.

Tubal ligation, known colloquially as getting your tubes tied, is the most common sterilization procedure for women and involves the closing of the fallopian tubes. These tubes have the dual job of delivering the sperm in semen to the egg, or ovum, and the egg to the uterus. They are not literally tied up, but often either surgically cut, clipped or cauterized. Both of these procedures are considered to be low risk and relatively safe, though unintended complications can arise, as they can in any medical procedure.

Why do people choose sterilization?

Sterilization is a form of birth control, and many people choose it for the same reasons that they would choose other forms of birth control- they do not want to have children. The difference between using sterilization as compared to other methods of birth control, such as condoms or the birth control pill, is the element of permanence of sterilization. Therefore, those who choose sterilization are certain that they do not want children, or do not want any more children. Knowing that there is a level of permanence also makes it easier for those who choose sterilization as birth control as there is less worry of unwanted pregnancies because of a missed pill or a torn condom.

There are several reasons why people want permanent birth control in the form of sterilization. As more women enter the workforce, some of them choose to be childless and focus on their careers. While some often have children at a later stage, others are choosing to forego having children altogether. Some families realize that having children is too expensive, or they can only afford to have a certain number of children. Some families or individuals choose to undergo sterilization to avoid passing on genetic defects. These families may choose to forego having children altogether, or to choose to use a donor sperm or egg. Some parents may have a child that is developmentally disabled and choose not to have more children in order to focus their energy and financial resources helping the one they have.

Sterilization and Medical Ethics

Whatever the reason may be, the rights for people to choose to undergo sterilization procedures falls under the medical ethics principle of patient autonomy. Patients are entitled to make reproductive health choices for themselves. Patient autonomy and personal consent are key in examining whether sterilization is ethical or not. Of course, if an individual is making an informed choice for himself or herself, then sterilization is ethical. But what happens when they are coerced to make a decision they don't want to, that could affect their ability to have children for the rest of their lives? And what if the coercion is stronger than mere encouragement and individuals are literally forced to undergo a procedure they don't want to or are ambivalent about?

It is clear that forced sterilization is unethical. It goes against patient autonomy and, by physically altering a person's body to be unable to reproduce, physicians performing the procedure may be considered to be causing harm to a patient. This goes against the principle of non-maleficence in medical ethics, so much so that the World Health Organization, UN Women, UN AIDS, The UN Family Planning Association, The UN Development Program, and UNICEF issued a joint statement in May 2014 condemning forced, coercive and other involuntary sterilizations.

Age and Patient Autonomy

While patient autonomy is paramount in medical ethics, even in the case of sterilization, physicians are morally obliged to provide the best medical advice to their patients for their overall health. This is enshrined in the principle of beneficence, which entails doing good for a patient. Given that sterilization is very difficult to reverse and is considered a permanent procedure, is it really in the best interest for a patient to be sterilized?

This is the question brought up by British medical ethicist and philosopher Piers Benn, who wrote about the topic in the British Medical Journal, along with Dr. Martin Lupton, an obstetrician and professor of medicine in London. The piece – entitled "Sterilization of Young, Competent, and Childless Adults" – explores just that. Benn and Dr. Lupton ask whether it is ethical to sterilize a young adult knowing the relative permanence of this procedure when there is a risk that they might change their minds about reproducing biologically as they get older.

Both authors state that there is a different risk in sterilizing a woman over 40 than there is sterilizing someone younger. They argue that the Hippocratic Oath states that one should do no harm to the patient. By performing a procedure that a patient may grow to regret, would a physician be harming a patient? They argue that if a physician has a strong belief that a patient could grow up to regret the procedure, they must balance the patient's current desires with their potential future needs and not follow through with performing the procedure. They recognize that this may be considered a paternalistic view that undermines the capacity and autonomy of the patient to decide for himself or herself. This is particularly relevant as few individuals, young or old, take the decision of sterilization lightly, given its permanence. Benn and Dr. Lupton argue that, even if everything is explained as above, it is not ethical to perform a sterilization on a younger patient.

Prejudice in Sterilization

Some governments have incentivized sterilization, particularly in countries that have high populations and struggle with population control. This does not mean that they have been egalitarian in going about it. It's clear that certain ethnic, religious or socioeconomic groups were being targeted by the campaigns. Even when the question of choice in terms of volunteerism was clear, the ethics of these situations was murky at best.

One example is the case of Singapore in the 1980s, where the government offered $5,000 to women who chose to be sterilized. The offer however, was not open to all women, but only to those whose families made less than $750 a month combined and had only achieved a certain level of education. Knowing these additional details, that the program only targeted the poor and uneducated, the program raises ethical concerns.

One could argue that the state, in this case, Singapore, was looking out for the best interests of the state and its citizens overall by curbing the population. It did, indeed, meet the goals that it set out to achieve by using this measure. It reduced the country's birth rate, infant mortality incidence, and female mortality rates. It also increased the number of women in the workforce and family income, among other things. Does the overall benefit outweigh individual choice in this case? And is the choice truly individual or was it taking advantage of the poor?

While Singapore could have been seen as giving some element of choice to women who chose to be sterilized, there are other instances when consent has not been given. A clear example of this was in India. India is a country that has struggled with overpopulation for decades. Because so much of the country is poor, many cannot afford birth control, and sterilization provides a one-time, cost effective solution. Because of this, sterilization incentives have been offered in the country for many years.

The Murky Ethics of Physician Incentives

In 1959, India began to offer doctors financial compensation to perform vasectomies on poor men. This clearly goes against medical ethics- doctors may perform these sterilization procedures on men potentially thinking not of a patient's best interests but of their own. This is in violation of the principle of medical ethical principle of non-maleficence. The men who received the vasectomies received money as well but, as in the case of Singapore, they were only available to the poor.

As in Singapore, the fertility rate dropped in India, but not fast enough for the government to meet its objectives in terms of population control. The situation worsened during the 21 months between 1975 and 1977 when India was under authoritarian rule during the regime of Prime Minister Indira Gandhi. This period of time was known as "The Emergency." In 1976, the emergency government regime decided that it needed to take more drastic steps to curb India's rapidly growing population problem. The government decided to put in some very unpopular policies that included compulsory sterilization. Not only did these take away patient autonomy, they also took place in "sterilization camps" that focused on speed and not on safety, resulting in numerous post-procedural complications. The harm done to patients – whether for a doctor's personal gain or otherwise – was a clear violation of the ethical principle of non-maleficence.

Unintended Consequences of Sterilization

While population rates can drop as a result of sterilization and this can improve society overall, forced sterilization can result in more ethical problems beyond the obvious ones related to patient autonomy and non-maleficence. In the case of India as described above and also in China through its one child policy, encouraging people – whether by force or voluntarily – to limit the number of children resulted in citizens selecting to favor male children. This led to female feticide, or selective abortions of female fetuses, and infanticide, or murder of newborn baby girls. It also led to sterilization being chosen only after people had a male child. The result of murder, neglect, and sterilization has led to uneven male to female population ratios in certain countries and a host of associated social problems related to this skewed gender ratio. Economist and Nobel laureate Amartya Sen has estimated that over one hundred million women are missing from the World's population, mostly in the Middle East, North Africa, and Asia. This is based on his analysis of the skewed gender ratio in these regions compared with the natural ratio that is expected.

Sterilization in the United States

State backed sterilization programs also occurred in the United States. Dr. Susan P. Raine, who is both a lawyer and a physician, wrote a piece for the American Medical Association Journal of Ethics in 2012 where she explored the unintended consequences of sterilization in the United States through the Federal Sterilization Policy.

Eugenics

Dr. Raine argues that in order to understand these consequences, one needs to understand the concept of eugenics. Basically explained, eugenics refers to facilitating and allowing reproduction amongst only the most fit and desirable in society with the intention of creating a better society overall.

In 1907, Indiana passed a law that allowed for sterilization for certain inmates in state institutions, including those with mental issues, convicted rapists and repeat criminals. Virginia followed suit in 1924. It passed a law that stated that those who had mental issues – specifically, called "mentally defective" – were legally allowed to be sterilized by force. This legal provision applied to women and men and was considered to be for the betterment of society. The idea was that if sterilized before being discharged, these individuals would be able to look after themselves better. There was also concern that their mental health issues were hereditary. By allowing for their sterilization, the law would diminish the risk of an increased number of mentally unwell residents of the state in future generations.

These number of states allowing for forced sterilizations grew after the Virginia law was upheld by the Supreme Court. In fact, by 1931, 30 states allowed for these forced sterilizations, something that Dr. Raine calls "eugenic laws." She argued that they discriminated against "some of the most vulnerable members of society." In the 1940s, attitudes towards eugenics had changed. Society recognized the practice as being particularly unfair to the economically and socially marginalized. Moreover, science showed that eugenics did not achieve the goal that it had set out to in terms of creating a certain kind of society. The Nazi genocide and holocaust of the 1930's and 40's also painted these laws and practices in a new light. Most states made the practice of forced sterilization illegal by the 1950s. Some estimate the number of forced sterilizations that had taken place by this time had risen as high as sixty thousand individuals.

While state laws addressed forced sterilizations, it took the federal courts well over twenty years to catch up. It was only in 1979 that the federal government created legal protections for those undergoing federally funded sterilization, requiring clear consent forms as well as proof that the individuals were competent and of sound mind enough to make this decision. Time protection measures, or waiting periods, were also put into place to ensure that those undergoing the procedure had thought about it and were not being taken advantage of. For example, consent forms were required to be signed and attested no less than thirty days before the procedure, but also no more than one hundred and eighty days from it.

By ensuring that the person was willing and able to consent to sterilization, the state was fulfilling the principle of personal autonomy. A woman or man's body is his or her own, and a decision as permanent as sterilization must be one that he or she makes willingly and is mentally competent to make.

The law, however, created a difference in treatment and procedures for those under federally funded programs and those who pay privately or through insurance. This brings about the question of whether it is ethically correct that an individual should be treated differently based on their method of medical funding. For example, while federally funded sterilizations required a letter of consent and the like, there was no such requirement for those paying privately: they could have the procedure done immediately, and without any such protections to ensure their personal autonomy was being considered in this decision. On the flipside, should a woman going through federally funded invasive surgery decide that she would like a sterilization at the same time to minimize risk and impact on her body, she would not be able to do so unless her forms had been filled and validated at least 30 days prior to the procedure.

Dr. Raine argues that the unintended consequences of the Federal Sterilization Policy are that, aside from creating different medical rules for the haves and have nots, it has also prevented those who most need sterilization from getting the procedure. She demonstrates that those who are poor may have forgotten the papers or lack the funding and wherewithal to have them validated. These women may already have limited access to birth control and find themselves with unwanted pregnancies, which may put additional financial pressure on them. She argues that it is ironic that while trying to give them more reproductive freedom and patient autonomy, these additional requirements may actually be curbing their patient autonomy.

Donation of Sperm and Eggs

This section will discuss the donation of sperm and eggs. As we highlighted at the beginning of the chapter, as technology becomes more advanced, new ethical issues arise. Parents are choosing to become parents at a later age, as they are marrying later due to pursuing educational or career goals. More women are participating in the workforce, and they may choose to delay having children until they feel more established in their careers. The acceptance by society of single gender families has created a demand for donated sperm and eggs. And there are also more single parent families, which sometimes require donation of sperm or eggs in order to create a baby, most often using in vitro fertilization, also known by the acronym IVF. These technological advances are welcomed by many who, prior to their discovery, only had the option of adoption if they wished to have a child. Adoption agencies have historically discriminated against same sex or single parent adoptions in the past, so when IVF technology developed it delivered a service with significant market demand.

In addition to providing an option for those who were perhaps biologically too old or single parents, IVF technology and specifically egg and sperm donation allow those who are afraid of passing on genetic disorders to still have a baby with a biological link to the other parent. Again, adoption would have been the only other option.

Despite all the positives, there are several ethical issues related to the donation of sperm and eggs, particularly considering that sometimes these are not donated but purchased. This has created a market, sometimes legitimate, and sometimes underground, for those desperately wanting to have children.

Adding to the dilemma of both egg and sperm donation, there are few laws governing this issue. Instead, there are guidelines on the process created by the American Society for Reproductive Medicine and the US Food and Drug Administration. These remain guidelines however, meaning that they are suggestions as opposed to legally binding conditions.

Is this a rich person's problem?

Finding an egg from another woman and having it implanted in another person's body can be a painful and extremely expensive process. It is not as easy to extract an egg as it is to get donor sperm for obvious biological reasons. Female egg donors must first undergo treatment with a hormonal medication to hyper stimulate their ovaries into producing several eggs. Side effects of these medications include allergic reactions, menopause like symptoms, and abdominal swelling. The ovarian stimulation can rarely cause a condition known as ovarian torsion, which can lead to permanent loss of ovarian function. Donors must then undergo a surgical procedure to extract the eggs from their bodies. One study estimated the rate of complications following this surgical procedure to be around two percent. Egg donors may spend over sixty hours of their time through this process in addition to the risks they face taking the medications and undergoing the surgical procedure itself.

On top of all this, the term donor egg can also be misleading. While in some cases family members step in to donate their own eggs, many women have to literally purchase an egg from a stranger, pay this person's medical bills as well as their own costs, and offer a hefty fee to the donor- who might be better described as a seller. None of this comes cheap.

One obvious ethical dilemma arises from this- purchasing or even receiving a donated egg from another woman and implanting it in one's body is so expensive that it is only a problem for the rich. Many women do not even consider the process because the cost is prohibitive, and it is usually not covered by health insurers. With this perspective in mind, only women or families of means have the option to go through this procedure.

While some women may donate eggs out of a motivation to help couples in need, the flip side of this argument is that the women who sell their eggs are more likely to be economically disadvantaged or struggling. A study showed that forty five percent of the egg donors in the US were students. The average payment for donations was $4,000 per donation, but can reach as high as $15,000. Egg removal is not without risks as well. A woman who might be financially stressed may feel as if she has no other choice but to go through with it in order to pay her bills or secure resources for herself or her family.

Donor's Rights Versus Recipient's Rights

It can be argued that egg purchasing is much like organ purchasing – but that is illegal. What are the ethical implications of buying one body part and not the other? Eggs, though finite in quantity, are much more numerous than organs like the kidneys, which are a popular item on the black market. Still, there is an underground trade in body parts. It is to avoid such issues and make the process more ethical that many countries do not allow for payment for donors. In the countries that do allow payment, it is said that the payment is not for the eggs, but rather for the donor going through the medical process of donation and egg retrieval.

In the United States, there is no cap on fees for a donor, which means that the compensation can change depending on supply and demand. In the European Union compensation for egg donation is capped at approximately $1,500. The results of this can be unfair- in Spain, for example, it means that only the poorest are willing to go through the process. What do you think is fair in this situation?

In addition, brokers and fertility agencies may be involved in the facilitation of egg donation. This means that they operate with profits in mind, and that they are capitalizing on other people's desires to have children. It also means that the safety protocols of clinics vary from facility to facility. While some clinics provide high quality and safe services, others are not significantly concerned about safety as much as they are about their own profits. No studies exist on the long-term effects of egg donation.

The Law on Egg Donation

In the United States, in addition to the medical fees, recipients are encouraged to hire lawyers in order to draw up clear contracts stating that the donors have no legal rights to the embryos and later children that may occur as a result of the donation. This also serves to protect the donors from any responsibilities – financial or otherwise – with respect to the embryo and child. These agreements are known as egg donor contracts.

Anonymity Versus Meeting the Donor

In the United States, parents have the option either to meet the egg donor, or to keep the process anonymous. The process can also be semi-anonymous, where the recipients are able to see photographs of the donor and her family. In the semi-anonymous case, the donors are also able to provide personal and medical records.

One can argue that semi-anonymous and anonymous methods fall under patient autonomy from the perspective of the recipient, as it would allow them to make the best decision in terms of who they wish to have as a child. For example, it can be incredibly painful for women not to be able to biologically reproduce. By seeking a donor that appears to have this ability and has a similar appearance, there is some comfort in knowing their child, though not biologically theirs, may resemble them and also have the ability to reproduce themselves. Parents essentially can choose a "designer baby" based on the physical characteristics of the donor, a practice reminiscent of historical eugenics movements.

Sperm Donation

Sperm are a lot easier to donate than eggs, as we touched upon earlier, and the process is of little risk to the donor. Like egg donation, sperm donation can be done privately, with a friend or family member – say, the brother of the male spouse in a couple – donating sperm. It can also be done through a sperm bank.

Unlike egg donation, sperm donation and the subsequent fertilization can be done at home either through sexual intercourse with the donor or a "turkey baster" technique. This makes it a much more affordable option than egg donation because medical intervention is not necessarily required for insemination. Even when it is, the costs of sperm donations are much lower and also much less taxing on the donor's body. Some countries, like Canada, do not allow payment for sperm donation. As a result, Canada has a shortage of sperm in sperm banks.

As in the case of egg donation, the reasons for sperm donation are much the same- either single or same sex parents hope to have a child, to avoid passing on of genetic diseases or mutations, or the inability of the recipient couple to biologically reproduce.

Donor's Rights in Sperm Donation

A sperm donor is similar to an egg donor in that legal contracts can rule out any rights and obligations to offspring produced through donated sperm. This is all subject to proper legal documentation. Because sperm is so much easier to donate than eggs and the process can be done without medical intervention, some sperm donors may find themselves liable for the children produced using their sperm. This is known as private or "directed" donation. For this reason, it is important for those who wish to remain out of the child's life to have proper legal documentation in place.

One may think that those who deal with sperm agencies, more commonly known as sperm banks, would have greater protection, but that's not always the case. There have been cases against sperm agencies for irregularity. Though donors may often be young men taking this situation lightly, they should in fact carefully consider all legal obligations before making a donation.

With genetic testing available over the internet these days, offspring may be able to track down their sperm donors, even if the donations were done anonymously. This is another ethical dilemma to consider when making a donation.

All things considered, egg and sperm donation do not come without ethical, legal, and medical risks, both for the donor and the recipient. All parties must be very clear where they stand legally and morally before making such an important decision.

Key Takeaways

- Reproductive health ethics hare continuously affected by social change and advancements in technology.

- Abortion refers to elective termination of a pregnancy. Those who are against abortion fall into the "pro-life" camp, whereas those who are for women having the right to choose are called, appropriately, "pro-choice."

- Abortion continues to be an ethical dilemma as guidance from the principles of autonomy and nonmaleficence are conflicting depending on underlying points of view.

- Being pro-choice meant that doctors prioritized a woman's right to govern her own body, which falls under respect for patient autonomy.

- Those who believe that life begins at conception clearly are at a conundrum when looking at a mother's health versus that of her fetus, and have to balance the idea of beneficence of the mother with that of non-maleficence towards the fetus.

- In the early 1900's, it is estimated that pro-choice physicians were performing 800,000 abortions a year. Many women who didn't have access to legal abortions or clandestine abortions in a physician's office however, were forced to undergo dangerous illegal ones.

- In 1972 the Supreme Court ruling Roe vs Wade allowed for access to abortion within the first trimester or twelve weeks of a fetus' existence. After this period, the court said a woman could still have access to abortion if the mother's life or health was in any danger.

- Maternal fetal conflict occurs when the health or interests of the mother are in conflict with the needs of the growing fetus. When deciding whether or not a mother's rights trump those of a fetus, similar ethical issues arise to the case of abortion. This is because there is still a lot of debate as to when a fetus becomes a person and has rights of their own.

- Maternal fetal conflict is complicated in cases where mothers refuse treatments on religious grounds. State laws do not allow pregnant women to be forced to go undergo a medical treatment if they refuse due to religious reasons. They say that not one but two ethical rules are being broken by doing so: a woman's right to patient autonomy as well as her human right to practice a religion.

- Sterilization refers to a number of medical techniques, many of which differ depending on the sex of the patient that leaves an individual unable to biologically reproduce. Sterilization can be permanent or reversible.

- Patient autonomy and personal consent are key in examining whether sterilization is ethical or not. If an individual is making an informed choice for himself or herself, then sterilization is ethical. If they are being coerced or tricked in to the procedure, then it is an unethical practice.

- Eugenics refers to facilitating and allowing reproduction amongst only the most fit and desirable in society with the intention of creating a better society overall. Eugenics was often used as a justification to forcibly sterilize prison inmates, the mentally ill, and marginalized social groups.

- Egg and sperm donation for in vitro fertilization has created new ethical dilemmas associated with this technology. In many cases, the eggs or sperm are purchased, and once cells are turned into commodities, they may be subject to market forces of supply and demand and price variability.

- Egg donation in particular is fraught with ethical issues as the donors often volunteer due to financial hardship. They may face potential side effects and complications from the medications and surgical procedure associated with the egg donation process.

Review Questions

1. Which of the following social changes has affected reproductive health ethics over the past several decades?
   a. Technological advancements opening new reproductive health options
   b. Legal and regulatory challenges
   c. Changing family structure
   d. All of the above

Answer: d. All of the above have impacted reproductive health ethics. Women are choosing to have children at a later age, and what families look like has evolved. Changes in reproductive technology have brought about exciting new methods available for those interested in being parents, to whom being pregnant or having a biological child would have been impossible in the past.

2. Proponents of legal abortion are usually referred to as what movement?
   a. Pro Abortion
   b. Pro Life
   c. Pro Choice
   d. Anti Regulation

Answer: c. Those who are against abortion fall into the "pro-life" camp, whereas those who are for women having the right to choose are called, appropriately, "pro-choice." For doctors, being pro-choice means that they prioritize a woman's right to govern her own body, which falls under respect for patient autonomy. In the case of pregnancy that could be dangerous or even fatal for a mother, doctors would be performing a life-saving procedure.

3. During the years when abortion was illegal, certain states permitted the practice under exceptional circumstances. These exceptions included which of the following?

a. Rape

b. Incest

c. Danger to the mother

d. All of the above

Answer: d. During the years when abortion was illegal, some states outlined exceptional circumstances that allowed for the practice to be performed. These circumstances included pregnancy as a result of rape or incest and also when the mother's life was in danger. In this latter case, it was agreed in these locations that the ideal of beneficence to the mother outweighed the non-maleficence to the fetus.

4. The ABCL founded by Margaret Sanger is the precursor to what modern organization?

a. National Organization for Women

b. Planned Parenthood

c. The Junior League

d. International Women's Health Coalition

Answer: b. The American Birth Control League or ABCL was an organization dedicated to pushing for the creation and promotion of birth control clinics. It's founder, Margaret Sanger, believed that women had the right to control their own fertility, and this included access to abortion. In 1942, the ABCL went on to become the Planned Parenthood Federation of America.

5. The case of Gerri Santoro highlighted what consequence of the criminalization of abortion?

a. High cost of illegal abortions

b. Injustice of having to travel abroad for an abortion

c. Danger of obtaining illegal abortions

d. All of the above

Answer: c. Many women who didn't have access to legal abortions or clandestine abortions in a physician's office, were forced to undergo dangerous illegal ones. These were often conducted by unscrupulous characters in unsanitary conditions and could result in extreme illness or death. Gerri Santoro also became a key figure in the pro-choice movement when she died due to complications from an illegal abortion in 1964. This galvanized women to train to perform safe abortions themselves, even though they were still illegal at the time.

6. What year did the Roe v Wade verdict legalize abortion in the United States?
    a. 1950
    b. 1962
    c. 1973
    d. 1979

Answer: c. Roe vs Wade was a legal ruling that remains synonymous with the battle for women's right to abortion in the United States. The landmark decision by the United States Supreme Court in 1973 ruled in favor of a woman's rights to an abortion. In their decision, Supreme Court justices cited the fourteenth amendment of the Constitution, which cited a woman's right to privacy.

7. Which of the following is an example of maternal fetal conflict?
    a. Miscarriage
    b. Retained products of conception after childbirth
    c. Woman uses heroin during pregnancy
    d. All of the above

Answer: c. Maternal fetal conflict occurs when the health or interests of the mother are in conflict with the needs of the growing fetus. So the desire of the mother to use heroin conflicts with the health status of the fetus, who will be born addicted to opiates.

8. The court case *In re Fetus Brown* grappled with what ethical dilemma?
    a. Maternal religious beliefs
    b. Sterilization
    c. Egg donation
    d. Surrogacy

Answer: a. *In re Fetus Brown* dealt with the issue of maternal religious beliefs. The case occurred when a pregnant woman refused a potentially lifesaving blood transfusion due to a religious objection to the practice.

9. Which of the following is not a form of sterilization?
    a. Tubal ligation
    b. Oral contraceptive pill
    c. Vasectomy
    d. Hysterectomy and oophorectomy

Answer: b. Oral contraceptives are considered temporary means of birth control. Sterilization refers to a number of medical techniques, many of which differ depending on the sex of the patient, that leave an individual unable to biologically reproduce.

10. What ethical issues are raised by sperm and egg donation?
    a. Anonymity of donors
    b. Donors usually economically disadvantaged
    c. Recipients usually economically elite
    d. All of the above

Answer: d. Sperm and egg donation raise numerous questions regarding the anonymity of the donor and related to the power dynamic between the wealthy recipient and the needy donor.

Chapter 5: End of Life Ethics

This chapter will discuss ethical issues around end of life care and will cover topics including advanced directives, withdrawal of medical treatment, medical futility, and physician assisted suicide. The topic is alluded to once again in the Hippocratic Oath, providing some initial guidance: *Most especially must I tread with care in matters of life and death. If it is given me to save a life, all thanks. But it may also be within my power to take a life; this awesome responsibility must be faced with great humbleness and awareness of my own frailty. Above all, I must not play at God.*

The advancement of medical science and technology have allowed treating physicians to prolong human life as never before. Oftentimes however, this technology is utilized without consideration of a patient's future meaningful recovery and independence from the life sustaining machines. While death is inevitable for us all, its timing is now, more than ever under the power of medical practitioners administering life prolonging treatments in health facilities.

Prior to the advent of intensive care facilities in hospitals in the 1950s and 60's, the majority of Americans died at home and only about one third died in hospital facilities. Today, the ratio has reversed with only 20% dying at home, and 80% dying in hospitals and nursing homes. These statistics reflect the increasing medicalization of death and dying and have a raised a new set of complex issues and decisions for patients, family members, and physicians alike.

The widespread availability of life prolonging medical technologies combined with the trend towards providing end of life care in a clinical, rather than home based, setting, present several ethical challenges for treating physicians. Physicians must consider the issue of patient autonomy and make a determination of what level of treatment a patient would desire. Oftentimes this decision must be made in a setting where the patient is unable to verbalize their own wishes due to dementia or as a consequence of their medical illness.

Similarly, physicians must weigh the principles of beneficence and non-maleficence against each other in these situations. Do they do good by providing medications to alleviate pain and allow a terminal patient to die peacefully? Or should any treatment hastening death be considered doing harm? Should they continue administering invasive and painful treatments and procedures to prolong life in cases of medical futility, or should they withdraw these treatments and focus instead on the quality of life during the patient's last days?

Advance Directives

If a patient is competent and has made their wishes known, it is the ethical duty of the treating physician to respect the boundaries of the patient's wishes following the principle of autonomy. Patients often express their preferences in advance of their illness by providing a written document known as an advanced directive.

These documents, also known as living wills, specify what actions a patient would like their health providers to take in different situations in the event that they are too ill to verbalize their own wishes. This document is often paired with a health care proxy document which names a person able to make these decisions for them if they are unable to do so.

These documents take many forms, but the five wishes document serves as an illustrative example. Firstly, this document asks patients to designate a medical decision maker in case they are incapacitated. Next, they select the types of treatments they would like administered in different situations. This could include or exclude intubation and mechanical ventilation, defibrillation, and chest compressions. Then they indicate their desired level of comfort and how they would like others to treat them at the end of their life. And finally the patient writes a message to their loved ones to be read at the time of their death.

It is important to distinguish living wills from do not resuscitate orders, or DNR's. While the living will is a legal document, the DNR is a medical order written by a physician. A physician can place a DNR order into the record after speaking with the patient, reviewing their living will, or discussing the situation with the patient's family members. When a DNR is in place, a resuscitation will not be attempted if the patient stops breathing or if their heart stops beating. Put another way, these patients will not be intubated and no chest compressions or defibrillation will be performed.

Withdrawal of Medical Treatment

While it is relatively easier to withhold treatments in cases where a patient has expressed their wishes verbally or in a legal document, the situation becomes more complicated when life sustaining treatments and procedures have already been initiated before a patient's wishes become known. This happens frequently when patients are intubated and placed on a mechanical ventilator by paramedics or upon arrival to the emergency room. Only later, when family members arrive with the patient's health records, do the care providers realize that the patient had an advanced directive requesting that they not be intubated in the case of respiratory failure.

Withdrawal of treatment could involve turning off a mechanical ventilator, stopping intravenous fluids or enteral nutrition, or cancelling a surgical procedure. Withdrawal of treatment can be performed in cases where continuation of these treatments would be considered medically futile. This determination should be made in cooperation with the entire medical care team and the patient's family, as there is no strict legal or medical definition of futility.

Common scenarios where providers and family members are likely to agree on the issue of futility include brain death and in cases where a patient is unlikely to survive an intervention like a surgical procedure. Physicians are not ethically required to provide or continue treatments when there is no reasonable expectation that these treatments will be helpful. Nevertheless, decisions to withdraw or withhold care should be made in partnership with the patient, if possible, and their family members before a final decision is made.

Physician Assisted Suicide

Physician assisted suicide is defined as a physician providing medications for a patient to end their own life. This could take the form of a prescription for a large dose of morphine or other sedative that the patient would ingest or inject themselves. This definition is in contrast to euthanasia, where a physician would not only prescribe the medication but also administer it. Euthanasia is currently only legally permitted in Belgium, the Netherlands, Columbia, and Luxemburg.

Proponents of physician assisted suicide consider the practice to be an extension of the physician's duty to alleviate suffering and respect a patient's autonomy. Physician assistance is often requested in cases of terminal illnesses when patients desire control over the time, circumstances, and level of pain surrounding their death.

Oregon is currently the only state in the United States that allows physician assisted suicide. Since the implementation of the state's death with dignity act in 1997, physicians have been permitted to prescribe a lethal dose of a medication to patients with a terminal illness. The illness must have progressed to a stage where the patient has less than six months to live, and a second physician must review the case before the medication is prescribed. The law also outlines safeguards evaluating potential physician conflicts of interest and requiring psychiatric screening of patients when a mental illness like depression is suspected.

Opponents of physician assisted suicide state that the practice violates the principle of non-maleficence. Put another way, the physician is using their medical expertise and training to directly cause the patient's death. To opponents, this practice is a violation of the Hippocratic Oath and is at odds with the fundamental characteristics of the doctor patient relationship. When legalized, they believe that it can jeopardize the rights of weak or marginalized individuals forced into ending their lives by unscrupulous family members or health providers. Opponents of the practice argue instead for improved palliative care, aggressive treatment of the symptoms of painful terminal illnesses, and maintaining patient comfort and dignity rather than prematurely ending their life.

Principle of Double Effect

A common scenario during end of life care is the administration of treatments that alleviate pain, but hasten death. These scenarios have a double effect, both good and bad. An example of this would be administering ever increasing doses of morphine to a patient with a terminal illness. The morphine may be needed to keep the patient comfortable and manage their pain. However, with each increase in does the medication maybe shortening the patient's life by suppressing their respiratory drive.

According to the principle of double effect such actions can be permissible if certain conditions are met. Firstly, the action must not contradict the ethical principle like beneficence and non-maleficence. Administering an analgesic to a patient in pain for example, is meant to improve the patient's condition not cause harm. Secondly the negative effects of the action is not the intent of the person and taking it, although it may be predicted. So the treating doctor does not intend for the medication to cause harm, although they understand the potential side effects. Finally, there is no other course of action that can be taken to achieve the good effect avoiding the bad effect.

This principle and specific case scenario is considered every day for many thousands of patients receiving hospice care. The purpose of hospice care is to alleviate pain at the end of life. This often involves administering high doses of pain medications. Suppression is not the intent of hospice providers, it is tolerated in order to provide the intended benefit to their patients.

- The advancement of medical science and technology have allowed treating physicians to prolong human life as never before. Physicians must consider the issue of patient autonomy and make a determination of what level of treatment a patient desires. Oftentimes this decision must be made in a setting where the patient is unable to verbalize their own wishes due to dementia or as a consequence of their medical illness.

- Patients often express their preferences in advance of their illness by providing a written document known as an advanced directive. These documents specify what actions a patient would like their health providers to take in different situations in the event that they are too ill to verbalize their own wishes.

- Living wills must be differentiated from do not resuscitate orders, or DNR's. While the living will is a legal document, the DNR is a medical order written by the physician. When a DNR is in place, a resuscitation will not be attempted if the patient stops breathing or if their heart stops beating.

- A physician can place a DNR order into the record after speaking with the patient, reviewing their living will, or discussing the situation with the patient's family members.

- Physicians are not ethically required to provide or continue treatments when there is no reasonable expectation that these treatments will be helpful. Nevertheless, decisions to withdraw or withhold care should be made in partnership with the patient, if possible, and their family members before a final decision is made.

- Physician assisted suicide is defined as a physician providing medications for a patient to end their own life. This could take the form of a prescription for a large dose of morphine or other sedative that the patient would ingest or inject themselves.

- Oregon is currently the only state in the United States that allows physician assisted suicide. Since the implementation of the state's death with dignity act in 1997, physicians have been permitted to prescribe a lethal dose of a medication to patients with a terminal illness.

- Proponents of physician assisted suicide consider the practice to be an extension of the physician's duty to alleviate suffering and respect a patient's autonomy.

- Opponents of physician assisted suicide state that the practice violates the principle of non-maleficence by directly causing the patient's death.

- The definition of physician assisted suicide is in contrast to euthanasia, where a physician would not only prescribe the medication but also administer it. Euthanasia is currently only legally permitted in Belgium, the Netherlands, Columbia, and Luxemburg.

Review Questions

1. Prior to the advent of intensive care medicine in the 1950's and 1960's, what percentage of people in the United States died in a hospital?
   a. 30%
   b. 50%
   c. 70%
   d. 80%

Answer: a. Prior to the advent of intensive care facilities in hospitals in the 1950s and 60's, the majority of Americans died at home and only about one third died in hospital facilities. Today, the ratio has reversed with only 20% dying at home, and 80% dying in hospitals and nursing homes.

2. Today, what percentage of people in the United States die in a hospital or other health facility?
   a. 30%
   b. 50%
   c. 70%
   d. 80%

Answer: d. Prior to the advent of intensive care facilities in hospitals in the 1950s and 60's, the majority of Americans died at home and only about one third died in hospital facilities. Today, the ratio has reversed with only 20% dying at home, and 80% dying in hospitals and nursing homes.

3. Which of the following principles of medical ethics are relevant to the issue of end of life care?
    a. Autonomy
    b. Beneficence
    c. Non maleficence
    d. All of the above

Answer: d. Physicians must consider the issue of patient autonomy and make a determination of what level of treatment a patient would desire. They must also keep in mind the principles of beneficence and non-maleficence when deciding on what treatments are reasonable in cases of terminal illnesses and medical futility.

4. Which of the following is a definition of an advanced directive?
    a. A document which names a person able to make decisions for the patient if they are unable to do so
    b. A legal document specifying what actions a patient would like their health providers to take in different situations
    c. A medical order written by the physician that preempts resuscitation if the patient stops breathing or if their heart stops beating
    d. All of the above

Answer: b. An advanced directive is a legal document specifying what actions a patient would like their health providers to take in different situations.

5. Which of the following is a definition of a health care proxy?
    a. A document which names a person able to make decisions for the patient if they are unable to do so

b. A legal document specifying what actions a patient would like their health providers to take in different situations

c. A medical order written by the physician that preempts resuscitation if the patient stops breathing or if their heart stops beating

d. All of the above

Answer: a. A health care proxy is a document which names a person able to make decisions for the patient if they are unable to do so.

6. Which of the following is a definition of do not resuscitate order?

a. A document which names a person able to make decisions for the patient if they are unable to do so

b. A legal document specifying what actions a patient would like their health providers to take in different situations

c. A medical order written by the physician that preempts resuscitation if the patient stops breathing or if their heart stops beating

d. All of the above

Answer: c. A medical order written by the physician that preempts resuscitation if the patient stops breathing or if their heart stops beating. Put another way, these patients will not be intubated and no chest compressions or defibrillation will be performed.

7. What is the legal definition of medical futility?

a. A terminal illness at any stage

b. A terminal illness at the final stage

c. A severe life threatening medical condition or injury

d. There is no legal definition of medical futility

Answer: d. Withdrawal of treatment can be performed in cases where continuation of these treatments would be considered medically futile. This determination should be made in cooperation with the entire medical care team and the patient's family, as there is no strict legal or medical definition of futility.

8. In what state of the United States is physician assisted suicide legal?

a. Alabama

b. Florida

c. Oregon

d. Virginia

Answer: c. Oregon is currently the only state in the United States that allows a physician assisted suicide. Since the implementation of the state's death with dignity act in 1997, physicians have been permitted to prescribe a lethal dose of a medication to patients with a terminal illness. The illness must have progressed to a stage where the patient has less than six months to live, and a second physician must review the case before the medication is prescribed.

9. What is the definition of physician assisted suicide?

a. A physician administers a lethal dose of a medication

b. A physician prescribes a lethal dose of a medication

c. A physician advises a patient to end their life

d. All of the above

Answer: b. Physician assisted suicide is defined as a physician providing medications for a patient to end their own life. This could take the form a prescription for a large dose of morphine or other sedative that the patient would ingest or inject themselves. This definition is in contrast to euthanasia, where a physician would not only prescribe the medication but also administer it.

10. What are common arguments against the practice of physician assisted suicide?

a. Violates the physician patient relationship

b. Can be used to violate the rights of poor or marginalized individuals

c. Often used instead of improving palliative care

d. All of the above

Answer: d. Opponents of physician assisted suicide state that the practice violates the principle of non-maleficence by directly causing the patient's death. To opponents, the practice is a violation of the Hippocratic Oath and is at odds with the fundamental characteristics of the doctor patient relationship. When legalized, they believe that it can jeopardize the rights of weak or marginalized individuals forced into ending their lives by unscrupulous family members or health providers. Opponents of the practice argue instead for improved palliative care, aggressive treatment of the symptoms of painful terminal illnesses, and maintaining patient comfort and dignity rather than prematurely ending their life.

Chapter 6: Physician Patient Relationship

This chapter will discuss the physician patient relationship and highlight ways in which it is unique and unlike other professions. The Hippocratic Oath features a clause specific to this relationship: *I will remember that I remain a member of society, with special obligations to all my fellow human beings, those sound of mind and body as well as the infirm.*

The special doctor patient relationship allows for the necessary trust to exist to diagnose disease and administer treatments. Doctors have unique obligations towards their patients that form the basis of this trust. These obligations include a fiduciary relationship, confidentiality, and honesty. In order to preserve and safeguard this relationship, doctors must submit themselves to heightened financial and personal scrutiny. This ensures that they are free from conflicts of interest or personal impairment. This scrutiny often comes at the time of medical license renewal or issuance or during the credentialing process at a new hospital. Doctors may have to submit themselves to drug testing and fingerprinting, or have to reveal any history of criminal charges or legal proceedings.

Certain relationships and interactions with clients that would be allowed for members of other professions are not permitted for physicians in order to maintain the doctor patient privilege. Examples include sexual relationships with patients and acceptance of lavish gifts in exchange for preferential treatment.

The doctor patient relationship also requires that physicians be open and honest when medical errors occur. Failure to do so jeopardizes not only individual relationships but trust and faith in the medical profession as a whole.

The doctor patient relationship ensures that doctors received the information, respect, and trust needed from the patient in order to effectively perform their duties. It also ensures that patients will adhere to treatment recommendations provided by their doctors. The general medical Council of United Kingdom summarized the doctor patient relationship in a pamphlet titled "what to expect from your doctor." The Council states that doctors should be expected to provide good care, keep their patients' safety in mind, use resources responsibly, help to train other health providers, and strive to be honest and trustworthy.

When does the relationship begin?

An important question to ask related to this topic is- when does the doctor patient relationship begin? This is both an ethical question and a legal one, as it determines when a doctor is expected to adhere to the principles, rules, and responsibilities required of them as the treating physician.

As a general rule, doctors can choose whether or not to enter into a doctor patient relationship with a person in need of care. Legal precedent has upheld this guideline. Physicians without a prior relationship with a patient can choose to provide treatment as a provider or they can refuse to do so. Physicians who have begun treatment, performed an examination, made a recommendation, or made a verbal agreement to take action as a doctor on call or consulting physician however, have in fact begun a care relationship so are obligated to continue care according to their responsibility as the treating physician. Of course, the right to refuse care does not apply to doctors working in an emergency room, who must treat all patients that come through the door. It is also not permitted to refuse treatment based on a personal characteristic of the patient as that would be defined as discrimination.

If a physician has begun to treat a patient and developed a doctor patient relationship as defined by both legal and ethical rules, they are not required to hold this responsibility in perpetuity. Doctors have the right to terminate their relationship under appropriate circumstances. Termination of the care relationship must occur in writing and with clear notification to the patient. The patient must be given ample time to find another provider, and the original provider could even provide referrals to other physicians who can provide the patient with appropriate care. If the doctor does not adhere to these guidelines when terminating the relationship, they may be accused of patient abandonment and be held liable for any associated damages.

Confidentiality

The issue of confidentiality has already been discussed in chapter three. Confidentiality is a core principle of the physician patient relationship and is mentioned in its own specific section of the Hippocratic Oath. Confidentiality aligns with a core value of medical ethics, justice. Justice here refers to the patient's right to be treated fairly in a safe and secure environment.

Physicians have an ethical duty to keep patient information confidential. Medical records can only be shared with the patient's permission. This confidentiality can be breached in the case of a few exceptions that have already been discussed. In brief, these include times when maintaining patient confidentiality could theoretically cause an individual or group harm unless breached. Examples of such circumstances include cases where there is suspected child abuse, mental illness when a patient is suicidal or homicidal, and reportable conditions where the physician is legally required to provide information.

The issue of confidentiality speaks to trust needed in the doctor patient relationship for medical care to be provided. Patients often must share private, intimate, potentially embarrassing personal details with their physician in order for the physician to provide adequate care. These issues can include sensitive reproductive, sexual health, psychiatric, or substance abuse issues.

A female patient with a complaint of abdominal pain for example, must trust her treating physician will keep her medical history confidential. If not, she might not feel comfortable revealing a sexual encounter that preceded the onset of her symptoms. If the treating physician is not trusted with this information, they might assume that her symptoms stem from a gastrointestinal issue and fail to diagnose a potentially dangerous gynecological infection like pelvic inflammatory disease.

A key feature of the doctor patient relationship is the concept of shared decision making. This means that both the doctor and the patient have a say in the treatment course, and that it is the duty of the physician to provide the right level of information on what options are available. This is also known as informed consent.

Informed consent relies on patients of sound mind with intact decision making capacity. These patients are provided with the appropriate knowledge of treatment options, the positive and negative consequences of each potential option, and costs and benefits associated with them. They must then be permitted to choose the option that best suits their values and desires, even if this choice contradicts the recommendation of a medical provider. An example of such a disagreement would be a case where a patient refuses a potentially lifesaving therapy, such as a blood transfusion, due to their religious beliefs.

Autonomy is the core value behind the concepts of informed consent and shared decision making in choosing medical treatment options. A patient's autonomy, or their personal right to decide to pursue or refuse treatment, can only be overruled in situations when their capacity is impaired. Examples of this impairment include intoxication, psychiatric illness, and dementia.

The concept of informed consent and shared decision making is in stark contrast to another approach to the doctor patient relationship that has been prevalent in previous eras, that of paternalism. Paternalism is defined as the practice of authority figures- like doctors, elders, leaders, and parents, making decisions on behalf of others in the name of those individuals' best interests. When paternalism was the norm in the practice of medicine, a doctor might withhold information from the patient in order to protect them from the trauma of knowing their prognosis. For example, they might not tell a frail, elderly patient that they had cancer in order to let them die a natural death. They might also make treatment decisions for patients based on what they thought would be best for them. Doctors in the past were even known to administer placebo treatments, or therapies that they knew to be without benefit, for the sole reason of comforting a patient and providing false hope.

Some medical ethicists argue that true informed consent and universal decision making is not possible and in many cases not desirable. First of all, they argue that complete understanding of medical nuances by the patient is nearly impossible. Medicine is a complex subject that takes years of study to truly understand. So how can a patient without a medical education ever hope to be truly informed about the treatment options presented to them? If a doctor attempted to provide medical information in the detail required to make an informed decision, these ethicists argue that they would leave the patient more confused than ever.

Secondly, opponents of informed consent argue that many patients may simply not want to know if they have a serious, terminal condition, or may be overwhelmed with the knowledge. Telling the truth in this situation might actually have a negative impact, which would go against the principle of non-maleficence. These patients might also prefer that their doctor take a paternalistic approach to their relationship and decide what is best for them, so refusing to fulfill that role disrespects the patient's autonomy to request that type of care. Additionally, they argue that placebos should be considered permissible despite their lack of a therapeutic effect. Placebos may have a psychological effect on the patient which makes them worthwhile according to the principle of beneficence.

Despite these arguments to the contrary, most modern medical ethical guidelines and regulations rely on the concept of informed consent and exceptions should only be made in rare circumstances, not as a general approach or practice style.

Fiduciary relationship

The concept of a so called fiduciary relationship is a helpful starting point when evaluating the physician patient relationship. The word fiduciary is defined as the trust between a person with power or responsibility, and a beneficiary with whom they interact. A person with power or responsibility can be referred to as a trustee or even a fiduciary. The beneficiary is usually in a disadvantaged position, with regard to power or knowledge, relative to the trustee. The trustee therefore has both a legal and ethical duty to act in the best interests of the beneficiary and to hold the interests of the beneficiary above their own personal motivations. This is known as the fiduciary duty and it requires the trustee to act free from conflicts of interest and personal motivations.

A recent law related to financial advisors in the United States, known as the fiduciary rule, provides a good example of this concept. The fiduciary rule designated all financial advisors that offer retirement planning advice as fiduciaries or trustees. This means that they are now required to clearly disclose any potential conflicts of interest in their retirement planning advice to their clients. Prior to the rule, these advisers were only required to offer investments according to the suitability standard. This meant that they could sell any investment that was suitable for a client's interests and needs. They could however hide the fact that they received commissions and bonuses related to the specific products that they recommended. Many argue that this practice was a conflict of interest and potentially harmful to individuals planning their future retirement. The argument states that these individuals were steered towards products like mutual funds, annuities, and bonds not because they were the best choices for their future but because the financial planner was making a profit off of them. According to the standards of the fiduciary rule, any commissions and bonuses related to all recommended products must be disclosed to the clients. The rule does not prevent such products from being offered, only that the benefit to the financial planner is disclosed up front. The purpose of this rule is to ensure that retirement planning focused financial advisors provide their clients with the best possible choices, not just choices that are good enough.

The definition of the fiduciary concept and the example of the fiduciary rule fit well with this discussion on the doctor patient relationship. Here, the physician is the responsible party and the patient is the beneficiary. There is clearly an inequality of power between physicians and their patients, since physicians alone have the medical knowledge that can address a patient's health care needs. They therefore have both a legal and ethical duty according to the definition of a fiduciary relationship.

In the health setting, the fiduciary relationship places several requirements on the trustee physician. A physician must be fully competent and accredited to undertake their duties. This means that they must have the proper training, licensure, and accreditation to provide the health care services that they offer. They should not offer advice or treatments outside of their scope of practice. This is known as the duty of competence. Next, doctors must provide and recommend treatments that are in patients' best interests, according to the beneficence principle. This is also known as the duty of good faith, and it also requires that physicians should charge reasonable fees for their services and not add additional services or costs in order to maximize billing proceeds. Doctors should never prescribe a treatment that goes against the best interest of their patient, which would violate the ethical duty on non-maleficence. This is known as the duty of loyalty. And finally, treatments that benefit the physician should not be pushed on the patient, even if they may be suitable for the purpose, unless they are the best potential option. Where possible, physicians should avoid potential conflicts of interest that could erode this fiduciary relationship such as selling medications that they also prescribe.

An interesting example of the fiduciary concept in health dates back to ancient Greece and was even referenced in the original text of the Hippocratic Oath. During the time of Hippocrates kidney and bladder stones, or *lithos*, were commonplace and many healers of the time would attempt to remove them using brutal and unrefined surgical procedures. Of course, these procedures were done in unsanitary conditions, without adequate anesthesia, and resulted in high complication and death rates. Hippocrates considered these procedures to be more harmful than beneficial, and he noted that the healers also acknowledged this fact. They nevertheless continued to carry out the practice out of personal self-interest since they could charge higher fees for more invasive procedures like this practice of "cutting for stone." According to the original Hippocratic Oath, healers would recite the following line-- "I will not use the knife, not even, verily, on sufferers from stone, but I will give place to such as are craftsmen therein." The phrase "cutting for stone" has, in recent years, been used as the title of a best-selling novel by physician author Abraham Verghese. The phrase is synonymous with physicians practicing outside of their scope and for placing personal interests ahead of those of their patients.

Conflicts of Interest

A conflict of interest is defined as an opportunity for a person to make personal profit from decisions they are making in their official capacity or profession. Examples from the field of medicine include a physician selling medications or products that they also recommend and prescribe. Even if the medication or product is effective, the obvious conflict of interest may damage the doctor patient relationship if the patient suspects that the doctor is prescribing the treatment to reap personal gain. Similarly, if the physician receives a kickback or incentive when they prescribe certain medications, a conflict of interest is present. Are they prescribing the medications because it is the best course of treatment for their patients? Or are they doing so in order to receive their commission?

Self-Care and Care for Family Members

Physicians providing treatment for themselves or family members is a contentious issue. Arguments against self-care or care for family members may seem obvious, yet physicians often make the mistake of crossing this ethical boundary. The primary reason to avoid this practice is due to the loss of objectivity, especially when treating family members. A treating physician may not be able to make tough decisions or recommendations when treating a close family member. Imagine a surgeon performing an operation on their own child. What would happen if a complication were to occur? Would the surgeon be able in such a circumstance to respond rationally to the complication and complete the surgery safely? Would they have the clinical detachment needed to manage a resuscitation if their child's heart stopped beating?

Also, from the perspective of a family member or relative, being treated by a health provider who is a family member is also problematic. What if the patient needs to disclose sensitive personal information, like a sexual or psychiatric history, that they have not felt comfortable sharing with other family members in the past?

Self-care is also a problematic issue. Although the biblical verse, "Physician, heal thyself," seems to open the door to self-care, the practice opens up a variety of ethical issues and potential complications. When a doctor writes a prescription or initiates a treatment course for themselves, they usually do not follow the usual process they employ when evaluating another patient. This process involves an in depth medical history, patient interview, and physical examination. When making decisions for oneself, there is an obvious loss of objectivity and clinical detachment. Self-care when related to narcotic prescriptions are particularly dangerous as they can lead to addiction. Addictive behaviors further cloud provider objectivity and can feed in to the spiral of abuse. Later in this chapter, we will discuss the issue of physicians impaired by addiction. This scenario can often arise as the result of an initial episode of self-care like writing a prescription for personal use. In the United States, narcotic prescription databases are monitored for instances where a physician is writing a prescription for their own personal use and this practice can lead to an investigation, censure, or loss of scheduled medication prescribing privileges.

The American Medical Association code of medical ethics has a specific clause dedicated to the issue of self-treatment and treatment of family members. According to the code, this practice raises concerns regarding patient autonomy, provider objectivity, and informed consent. According to the code, providers might feel pressured to provide care outside of their scope of practice. They might also shy away from asking important questions, like a sexual history, that might help them make a diagnosis. Similarly, patients may feel uncomfortable receiving care from a family member. They may not disclose sensitive information and they may feel unable to refuse care or request another provider. According to the AMA's ethical guideline, self-care and care for family members should only be provided in emergency situations or for short term or minor issues.

Impaired Physicians

This section will discuss the issue of physicians impaired by physical, mental, or substance related disorders. Physicians as a group suffer from the same challenges faced by the general population including alcohol and drug abuse, psychiatric illness, and dementia. Alcohol abuse is the most common cause of physician impairment. An estimated eight to twelve percent of physicians will suffer from some form of substance abuse during the course of their careers. Physicians working in the specialties of emergency medicine and anesthesiology are considered to have the highest risk of substance abuse compared with others. Impaired physicians place their patients at risk of medical errors and inappropriate care every day they continue to practice.

Physicians have an obligation to report colleagues they believe may be impaired to the appropriate authorities, including their department administration, hospital management, and state licensing board. Many states have license immunity programs where physicians who voluntary seek care for substance abuse are protected from losing their license if they follow a defined counseling and rehabilitation program.

Relationships with Patients

The doctor patient relationship is characterized by trust and an unequal power dynamic between the trained physician and the patient seeking care. As such, intimate relationships between doctors and their active patients are considered unethical. Several medical associations and boards consider the use of the doctor patient relationship to initiate a romantic relationship to be misconduct.

Opinions differ regarding doctors and their former patients. Some argue that such relationships may be permissible for specialists, urgent care providers, or emergency physicians who see a patient once and then terminate ongoing physician patient interaction. While some providers feel that these types of physicians should wait several months before initiating a romantic relationship, others argue that this is not necessary if the medical care relationship has been completed.

The ethics are even more unclear related to relationships with a patient's family members, and these cases should be evaluated on a case by case basis. The ethical response in these situations may depend on the level of interaction with the original patient in question. Were they treated for years for a serious chronic condition? Or were they treated briefly for a minor illness?

For rural physicians who are the only health providers in a region, it may be impossible to ban patient relationships altogether. These providers care for the entire local population, so it may be unreasonable to restrict them to only long distance relationships.

Gifts from Patients

There are no specific regulations related to accepting gifts from patients, but several professional societies provide helpful guidelines. Patients often express gratitude for the services they receive from their physicians. An estimated twenty percent of physicians report receiving gifts from patients. The ethical dilemma here arises related to lavish gifts, especially when a physician may be motivated or obligated to provide special treatment to the patient once they accept. For physicians who choose to accept a gift, the key is to not allow the care that they provide to be influenced moving forward.

Individual physicians have three choices when it comes to patient gifts. They can always accept gifts, never accept gifts, or accept gifts only under certain circumstances. The always approach is usually considered inappropriate. It is unethical for physicians to accept gifts that are extremely valuable or tied to future expectations of special services.

The never rule is ethical and it allows the physician to have a consistent approach. However, refusing gifts may harm the physician patient relationships and cause offense to patients who desire to express their gratitude.

Most physicians choose the conditional acceptance of gifts. When evaluating an individual gift, they can consider the motivation of the patient in giving it. Is the patient trying to secure preferential treatment? Is the gift itself an inappropriate item indicating romance or other intimacy? Is the gift extravagant? Physicians can also consider the timing of the gift. A gift given in late December for example, may be appropriate and in line with cultural norms of seasonal gift giving.

Medical Errors

The last section of this chapter will discuss medical errors. The practice of medicine is complex, and medical errors are inevitable. This can include a missed or incorrect diagnosis, a prescription error, or an inappropriate procedure. Medical errors are distinct from bad outcomes. An error would be if a patient receives a medication that they do not need. A bad outcome would be if they have an adverse reaction to a medication that they do need.

According to prevailing ethical standards and the need to preserve trust in the doctor patient relationship, all medical errors should be disclosed to patients immediately. Numerous studies have demonstrated that immediate disclosure along with an apology results in fewer malpractice lawsuits related to errors.

Key Takeaways

- Doctors have unique obligations towards their patients that form the basis of this trust. These obligations include a fiduciary relationship, confidentiality, and honesty. In order to preserve and safeguard this relationship, doctors must submit themselves to heightened financial and personal scrutiny. This ensures that they are free from conflicts of interest or personal impairment.

- If a physician has begun to treat a patient and developed a doctor patient relationship as defined by both legal and ethical rules, they are not required to hold this responsibility in perpetuity. Doctors have the right to terminate their relationship under appropriate circumstances. Termination of the care relationship must occur in writing and with clear notification to the patient

- Physicians have an ethical duty to keep patient information confidential. Medical records can only be shared with the patient's permission. This confidentiality can only be breached in the case of a few exceptions that have already been discussed. In brief, these include times when maintaining patient confidentiality could theoretically cause an individual or group harm unless breached. Examples of such circumstances include suspected child abuse, mental illness when a patient is suicidal or homicidal, and reportable conditions.

- Physicians should avoid conflicts of interest whenever possible. A conflict of interest is defined as an opportunity for a person to make personal profit from decisions they are making in their official capacity or profession. Examples from the field of medicine include a physician selling medications or products that they also recommend and prescribe.

- Physicians have an obligation to report colleagues they believe may be impaired to the appropriate authorities, including their department administration, hospital management, and state licensing board. Many states have license immunity programs where physicians who voluntary seek care for substance abuse are protected from losing their license if they follow a defined counseling and rehabilitation program.

- Certain relationships and interactions with clients that would be allowed for members of other professions are not permitted for physicians in order to maintain the doctor patient privilege. Examples include sexual relationships with patients and acceptance of lavish gifts in exchange for preferential treatment.

- All medical errors should be disclosed to patients immediately.

1. When does the doctor patient relationship begin?
   a. When a patient is referred to the doctor
   b. When a patient makes an appointment to see a doctor
   c. When a patient is examined and treated by a doctor
   d. All of the above

Answer: c. Physicians who have begun treatment, performed an examination, made a recommendation, or made a verbal agreement to take action as a doctor on call or consultant physician however, have in fact begun a care relationship so are obligated to continue care according to their responsibility as the treating physician.

2. In what situation must a doctor accept a doctor patient relationship?
   a. Emergency physician who sees a patient in the emergency room
   b. Specialist receives a consultation request when not on duty
   c. Patients calls physician office requesting appointment
   d. All of the above

Answer: a. The right to refuse care does not apply to doctors working in an emergency room, who must treat all potential patients. It is also not permitted to refuse treatment based on a personal characteristic of the patient as that would be defined as discrimination.

3. What is needed for a doctor to terminate a patient relationship?
   a. Written notification
   b. Patient provided time to find another provider
   c. Doctor provides referrals for other providers
   d. All of the above

Answer: d. If a physician has begun to treat a patient and developed a doctor patient relationship as defined by both legal and ethical rules, they are not required to hold this responsibility in perpetuity. Doctors have the right to terminate their relationship under appropriate circumstances. Termination of the care relationship must occur in writing and with clear notification to the patient. The patient must be given ample time to find another provider, and the original provider could even provide referrals to other physicians who can provide the patient with appropriate care. If the doctor does not adhere to these guidelines when terminating the relationship, they may be accused of patient abandonment and be held liable for any associated damages.

4. According to the fiduciary relationship, what role does the doctor play?
    a. Beneficiary
    b. Responsible party
    c. Executor
    d. All of the above

Answer: b. The definition of the fiduciary concept and the example of the fiduciary rule fit well with this discussion on the doctor patient relationship. Here, the physician is the responsible party and the patient is the beneficiary. There is clearly an inequality of power between physicians and their patients, since physicians alone have the medical knowledge that can address a patient's health care needs. They therefore have both a legal and ethical duty according to the definition of a fiduciary relationship.

5. Which of the following is a conflict of interest?
    a. Physician receives cash bonuses for referrals
    b. Physician runs their own laboratory
    c. Physician has their own pharmacy
    d. All of the above

Answer: d. A conflict of interest is defined as an opportunity for a person to make personal profit from decisions they are making in their official capacity or profession. Examples from the field of medicine include a physician selling medications or products that they also recommend and prescribe. Even if the medication or product is effective, the obvious conflict of interest may damage the doctor patient relationship if the patient suspects that the doctor is prescribing the treatment to reap personal gain. Similarly, if the physicians receives a kickback or incentive when they prescribe certain medications, a conflict of interest is present. Are they prescribing the medications because it is the best course of treatment for their patients? Or are they doing so in order to receive their commission.

their careers. Physicians working in the specialties of emergency medicine and anesthesiology are considered to have the highest risk of substance abuse compared with others. Impaired physicians place their patients at risk of medical errors and inappropriate care every day they continue to practice.

7. If a physician suspects a colleague is impaired, who can they make a report to?
   a. Department leaders
   b. Hospital Management
   c. State licensing board
   d. All of the above

Answer: d. Physicians have an obligation to report colleagues they believe may be impaired to the appropriate authorities, including their department administration, hospital management, and state licensing board. Many states have license immunity programs where physicians who voluntary seek care for substance abuse are protected from losing their license if they follow a defined counseling and rehabilitation program.

8. Under which circumstances might a doctor patient romantic relationship be permissible?
   a. Treatment was for minor illness
   b. Waiting period following treatment
   c. Following official termination of doctor patient relationship

d. All of the above

Answer: d. Opinions differ regarding doctors and their former patients. Some argue that such relationships may be permissible for specialists, urgent care providers, or emergency physicians who see a patient once and then terminate ongoing physician patient interaction. While some providers feel that these types of physicians should wait several months before initiating a romantic relationship, others argue that this is not necessary if the medical care relationship has been completed.

9. What characteristics of patient gifts to providers are concerning?
    a. Small gift during holiday season
    b. Lavish gift with expectation of special treatment
    c. Hand-written card expressing gratitude
    d. All of the above

Answer: b. Most physicians choose the conditional acceptance of gifts. When evaluating an individual gift, they can consider the motivation of the patient in giving it. Is the patient trying to secure preferential treatment? Is the gift itself an inappropriate item indicating romance or other intimacy? Is the gift extravagant? Physicians can also consider the timing of the gift. A gift given in late December for example, may be appropriate and in line with cultural norms of seasonal gift giving.

10. Immediate disclosure and apology for a medical error results in which of the following?
    a. Higher lawsuit incidence
    b. Disciplinary action
    c. Lower lawsuit incidence
    d. Low patient satisfaction scores

Answer: c. According to prevailing ethical standards and the need to preserve trust in the doctor patient relationship, all medical errors should be disclosed to patients immediately. Numerous studies have demonstrated that immediate disclosure along with an apology results in fewer malpractice lawsuits related to errors.

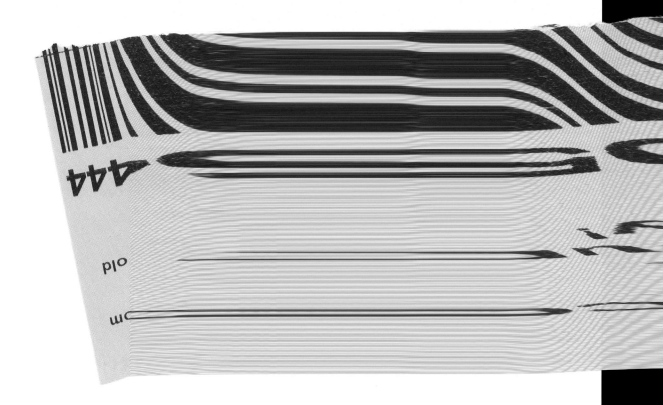

Chapter 7: Ethics in Global Health

This chapter will discuss the issue of global health ethics. Specifically, we will evaluate the history of global health and demonstrate the need to approach current and future initiatives with an ethical framework. Topics covered in this chapter include health as a human right, the social determinants of health, health worker brain drain, HIV/AIDS, the access to medicines debate, and short term medical volunteers. In this chapter we see how issues related to global health, international aid, and migration touch on the principles of justice, beneficence, non-maleficence, and autonomy. Whether you are personally involved in a global health initiative or you decide to support one with a charitable donation, it is important to keep these core principles in mind when evaluating decisions and actions.

Origin of Global Health and Development of Global Health Ethics

The journal Global Health Action recently published a study defining global health ethics as the process of employing concepts of morality to health challenges with global effects or requiring international coordination. While this is a simple definition, it nevertheless provides us with a good starting point. The practice of global health involves interactions across geographical boundaries and between different health systems, cultural perspectives, and communities. This poses a challenge for developing an ethical framework of analysis, as ethics is usually concerned with evaluating underlying values for each individual. Ultimately, the best approach in understanding global health ethics is to firstly understand its origin, development, and progression to the modern form it takes today.

First, we must look back to some of the origins of global health concerns – here we will discuss European imperialism during the 17th-18th centuries. The case of India demonstrates some of the negative economic impacts of the colonial era. During the 18th century, India was one of the richest regions on the globe, comprising 23 percent of the world's economy. Yet by the 19th century, its economy had been decimated. In the intervening century, the British colonial empire looted the subcontinent's raw materials and prevented the development of local manufacturing. The construction of the Indian railways helped imperial forces to transport and extract natural resources. Similar methods were employed in Africa, led by characters like Cecil Rhodes, prime minister of Cape Colony and founder of the DeBeers diamond cartel. His vision of a railroad and telegraph line from Cairo to Cape Town was not meant as a development initiative to help the people along its path. Instead it was planned as a way to extract the wealth of natural resources from the continent. This colonization era predominantly affected Africa and Asia, and in addition to Great Britain, involved France, Portugal, Spain, Holland, and Belgium.

When these European powers were arriving to these new, exotic shores they brought with them diseases and strains of bacteria that had never before been encountered. The native populations were exposed to disease such as smallpox, influenza, scarlet fever, and measles, which led to millions of deaths. The European colonizers themselves were also exposed to local diseases. These local diseases would later be referred to as "tropical diseases."

Colonizing forces began to bring along their own medical professionals during their colonial conquests in order to control the spread of diseases among their own forces. An article on the subject published in the Harvard College Global Health Review said it best-- "...global health's earliest efforts hark to a dark imperialistic history that tackled health concerns not out of benevolence or even of mutual benefit, but purely out of exploitation."

Even today global health has underlying political and economic incentives. The book "Health Care Under the Knife: Moving Beyond Capitalism for Our Health", by Howard Waitzkin, cites several examples of hospitals built in Indochina, North Africa, Iraq, and Afghanistan. While these were established under a veil of charitable medical services, they had the express purpose of gathering information on rebels and insurgents in the area. One recent example of that demonstrates the implications of approach occurred during the search for Osama bin Laden. The CIA created an elaborate vaccine campaign tracking samples of DNA in order to pinpoint family members and isolate his location. After these actions were revealed, polio vaccination efforts in the region were significantly affected, and some real vaccination health workers were murdered out of suspicion of ulterior motives.

Despite this recent case study, global health today is no longer dominated by exploitation and artifice. There are many positive examples from recent history where countries have joined forces and shared resources to fight diseases. Some examples include smallpox eradication in 1977, the ongoing global polio eradication initiative, and efforts to eradicate the infection that causes river blindness. The Carter Center for example, has made huge strides leading the global community in the eradication of both guinea worm and river blindness. It works by collaborating with local organizations and training local volunteers to carry out education and disease control interventions. Understanding the origin and motivations of past and current global health initiatives can provide us with an ethical framework to use when thinking about global health and perhaps even guidelines and standards that can steer us towards harm reduction and positive action.

Health as a Human Right

This section will discuss the concept of health as a human right. The discussion highlights one of the four core principles of medical ethics - justice. Good health and access to health care is today considered a basic human right. Achieving this around the world requires that resources be distributed equally and fairly. Nobody should suffer from a treatable disease while only a select few are being treated in sophisticated hospitals with high tech medical equipment.

In 1948 the international community codified the rights and freedoms of all individuals through the Universal Declaration of Human Rights. Forty eight countries collaborated on this historic document with the atrocities of World War Two still fresh on the global collective mind. The members of the United Nations agreed to thirty articles protecting human rights. To this day, the Universal Declaration of Human Rights continues to be utilized and implemented through treaties, national constitutions, and laws. Article twenty five of the Universal Declaration of Human Rights, highlights the importance of health as a human right. It states: "Everyone has the right to a standard of living adequate for the health and well-being of himself and of his family, including food, clothing, housing, and medical care and necessary social services, and the right to security in the event of unemployment, sickness, disability, widowhood, old age or other lack of livelihood in circumstances beyond his control." This and other articles of the declaration formed the basis of global development efforts to improve livelihoods in the years that followed.

Over thirty years later, in 1979, the Declaration of Alma Ata was launched at a global primary health care conference, further establishing the importance of accessible primary health care for every person in every country. The Declaration of Alma Ata set a target of health for all by 2000, and tasked the World Health Organization to lead the global community in achieving it. This set the agenda for global public health efforts, highlighting the need to tackle social, economic, and political challenges in order to improve the health of nations and regions.

The spirit of the Alma Ata Declaration continued to influence the global development agenda through the Millennium Development Goals which set social welfare targets between the year 2000 and 2015. Four of the eight total MDGs specifically focused on health. In 2016, the United Nations updated the agenda with the Sustainable Development Goals, or SDGs, setting goals and targets to achieve by 2030. SDG three focuses on ensuring healthy lives and wellbeing for all people of all ages, addressing topics such as maternal and child health, communicable diseases, substance abuse, reproductive health, and universal health care.

Global health today is inextricably linked to the concept of human rights. In 1948 it was included in the first global document on the subject, the Universal Declaration of Human Rights. Later it was codified in the Declaration of Alma Ata, which called on the global community to achieve health for all through primary health care. Today the Sustainable Development Goals set out concrete targets for the global community to achieve, calling for unprecedented levels of collaboration and resources to ensure success. These declarations of health as a fundamental right provide an ethical framework and justification to guide actions and strategies related to global health.

In order to achieve the goals for improved health around the world, attention must be directed not only to diseases, but also livelihoods and societies as a whole. This section will discuss the social determinants of health and how these factors are associated with good health. According to WHO the three core determinants of health are a person's social and economic environment, physical environment, and their individual characteristics and behaviors. These social determinants of health are all interconnected and affect one another. Social determinants of health touch on health as a human right and one of the core principles of medical ethics – justice. Justice requires that resources are distributed fairly around the world to create societies and environments that are healthy for the people living in them. From birth, these social determinants of health play a critical factor in the quality of life of an individual.

Social determinants of health include socio-economic status, education, access to health services, and physical environments. These are all interconnected and affect one another. For instance, studies show that individuals with lower income have lower quality health because of the lack of access to health services. Lower income is also associated with lower educational attainment because these individuals are unable to afford adequate education. Without education, many are stuck in low income jobs, and the resulting poverty in turn create a barrier to access critical health care services. Poverty is also connected to poor physical environments. These physical environments consist of polluted air and water and inadequate housing.

The greater a society's economic inequality, the greater the resulting health disparities. A recent study on global inequality showed that 8.6% of the global population own 86.5% of the global wealth. Inequities around the world and it specific regions are associated with unequal distributions of the resources households need be productive and healthy. The Universal Declaration of Human Rights states that everybody has the right to a standard of living adequate for the health and well-being of himself and his family. The social determinants of health help us understand how standards of living link to poor health.

Through the evaluation of social determinants of health in communities, we can develop clearer strategies to eradicating not only these social inequalities, but also the health effects associated with them.

Organizations and Global Aid

This section will focus on the role of development organizations and global aid, expanding on the issues of identifying and prioritizing the needs of communities and how organizations should act upon those needs. Global aid, also known as development assistance, is defined as the resources provided by governments or international agencies to support economic, political, social, and environmental development of a lower or middle-income country. While development assistance should be directed with the purpose of making life better in these countries and working towards the Sustainable Development Goals, in many cases it is offered for strategic or other political purposes without adequate oversight. One of the key ethical principles to keep in mind in this section is beneficence, which describes taking actions aimed at improving the general welfare of patients and keeping their best interests in mind. Many organizations in the past have failed to adhere to this ethical principle in their decision making related to their implementation strategies and resource allocation decisions. This failure often arises out of conflicting priorities and other complicated ethical dilemmas further discussed in this section.

The United States budget directs over thirty billion dollars to non-military foreign assistance, intended to benefit over three billion people around the world. Estimates of total global aid provided by wealthy countries is estimated to amount to over one hundred and forty billion dollars per year. Although these are huge numbers, oftentimes foreign aid is mismanaged and misdirected. It is sometimes spent without taking into account and prioritizing a receiving country's needs. Inefficiencies in aid spending can be perpetuated year upon year when the impact of aid is not evaluated.

A significant portion of development assistance is funds are directed towards non-governmental organizations, or NGO's. These NGO's can be international, based in the donor country, or based in the recipient country. They are tasked by the donors to implement projects that achieve the stated goals of the funding initiative. But the big question is- are these organizations really making a difference? Foreign aid is often directed towards public health projects that are ineffective. Many international organizations come to low income countries with a prearranged plan to eradicate malaria or treat HIV patients. Yet they fail to consult or communicate with people they are serving. One example arises from recent malaria eradication projects funded by the Global Fund, World Bank, and others which provided insecticide treated bed nets to prevent malaria. During the distribution of these nets, these organizations did not adequately explain the critical benefits associated with sleeping under these nets. A study in the Lake Victoria region of Tanzania, Uganda, and Kenya showed that 25% of the distributed nets were being used to fish. In other communities, bed nets have been used to protect chickens from hawks or make wedding dresses. This demonstrates the challenge of participatory development. Communities often prioritize different problems while organizations, despite their good intentions, have a different agenda in mind. The challenge for foreign organizations is to involve local people, according to the principle of participation, in project selection, planning, and implementation.

Development assistance agencies and NGO's face a dilemma when deciding how to allocate resources to global health. Which diseases should they focus on? How should programs be implemented?

We will dive deeper into the decision making process of resource allocation through the example The United States President's Emergency Plan for AIDs Relief, better known as PEPFAR. According to the United Nations and the WHO, the global death rate related to HIV and AIDS in 2003 was over three million people per year. This death rate was steadily climbing, as was heightened awareness of the disease's impact in poor countries. Motivated to do something to address the disease, President George W Bush and the US Congress established PEPFAR, a fifteen billion dollar project to be introduced in around 29 countries.

At first, there were many critics. Most notably USAID administrator Andrew Natsios, who stated that antiretroviral therapy in Africa would be ineffective since the region lacked trained doctors and adequate infrastructure. He went further by asserting that Africans could not follow a complicated treatment regimen due to their inability to tell time. Nevertheless, PEPFAR was launched and has proven to be hugely successful. PEPFAR now supports the treatment of over fifty million individuals in in Sub Saharan Africa. Prior to the program, fewer than fifty thousand in the region had access to treatment.

The PEPFAR example raises the ethical concern that development organizations in wealthy countries often make decisions on what course of action should be taken without full understanding of the needs, capacities, and opportunities in the countries they are supposed to be helping. Although these ethical issues commonly arise, they can be addressed once organizations start listening to community needs and involving communities in their decisions. It also poses another dilemma. For example, if a majority of rich country decision makers want funding for HIV prevention and only a few want resources directed towards HIV treatment – who decides how funds will be allocated? What if all resources were focused on preventing incidence of HIV and the population suffering from AIDS was neglected? These sorts of decisions require an ethical framework of analysis using the four principles of medical ethics: autonomy, justice, beneficence, and non-maleficence.

Short term medical experiences

This section will focus on short term medical experiences and their ethical implications. Short term medical experiences are when organizations and people come to countries for a few weeks or months to provide service and gain experience from working with tropical diseases. This is a particularly common practice for medical students and other trainees. A study found that of the 8,000 UK medical students who qualify as physicians every year, almost 40% of them will have spent at least 6 weeks on an elective in a developing country. Another study noted that benefits of participating in these medical experiences include increased knowledge of diverse syndromes and treatments, development of examination skills, and experience with different cultures and religions. Although there are many benefits for the trainees who participate in these short term medical experiences, one question to pose is if host countries are benefiting from these trips. Two core principles of medical ethics to keep in mind within this section is beneficence and justice. The principle of beneficence states that physicians must strive to act in the best interests of their patients, while justice requires respecting a patient's dignity, freedom, consent, equality, and fairness.

Many of the times through these medical trips, organizations bring medical equipment, supplies, and human resources to low income countries. Patients will seek out care from these medical missions often staffed by medical students and other trainees. As patients migrate towards the new, and often temporary, care facilities, existing clinics and healthcare facilities are underutilized and weakened. These facilities lose money because of the free services that are being provided by the mission teams. As institutions organize overseas medical experiences it is important for them to partner with and strengthen local, existing healthcare facilities.

Another consideration for overseas medical experiences is the long-term implications of treating patients in host countries. Many treatments take months of continuously administered medications and follow-up care, but with projects and staff only functional for a limited amount of time, many patients are only receiving parts of the needed care. Long term this leaves patients at a dangerous untreated state, often times with expired medications and suffering complications of medical procedures. Donations of time, supplies, and equipment should aim to have a long term and sustainable impact on local communities.

Although there are personal benefits in participating in medical trips within a foreign country, there are many ethical considerations to keep in mind. Many low-income countries have little regulation and oversight of accredited health professionals treating patients. Visitors should ask themselves if it is ethical for a medical trainee to go to another country and practice doing things on people that they would never be allowed to do in their home countries. These short term medical experiences are aimed to provide medical students with more hands-on experience and providing resources to vulnerable populations – but in reality, who is it really benefiting? Who bears the cost if a patient is hurt during the procedure or faces a complication months down the line? Is doing nothing sometimes better than doing something when that something has significant risks?

Brain Drain, Brain Gain, and Brain Circulation

This section will discuss the brain drain, brain gain, and brain circulation related to human resources for health. Many developing countries are suffering from the brain drain, which is defined as a migration of highly skilled health professionals from low income to high income countries. On the receiving end are the high-income countries who reap a brain gain from immigration of these highly skilled professionals. They get to enjoy the health and economic benefits of hosting these individuals without having to bear the cost of training them. Lastly, the brain circulation refers to a new phenomenon noted in recent years. Circulation involves an equal number of professionals migrating between low income and high-income countries and back again. This section will delve deeper into the government policies and ethical dilemmas involved in this movement of skilled labor.

High income countries have an increasing demand for health care professionals because of their aging population demographics. A recent study noted that the world's population over the age of sixty is expected to grow by fifty six percent by the year 2030, amounting to over 1.5 billion people. This rapidly aging population is due to several factors, most notably technological advancements able to prolong life. Because of the inevitability of disease in older individuals, we see an increasing demand for health care services and a strain on health care systems all over the world. In order to meet this demand, immigration policies in wealthy countries are often aimed at attracting highly skilled professionals. A study by Global Health Action shows that in Ireland, over thirty five percent of immigrants consisted of foreign trained nurses or doctors.

While high income countries reap benefits from these migrants, low income countries consequently suffer from shortages of skilled doctors and nurses. According to a recent article published in the international journal of gynecology and obstetrics, poor countries spend over five hundred million dollars annually training health professionals. When these health professionals leave their home country in pursuit of better working conditions, safety, and opportunities, the resources invested in them by their home countries is lost. Sub-Saharan Africa bears the overwhelming majority of these costs. While it is home to only ten percent of the World's population, it has over twenty five percent of the global burden of disease. Yet every year an estimated twenty-three thousand qualified academic professionals migrate to the US, Europe, and other high-income regions. This loss comes at a hefty price- contributing to low doctor to patient ratios, high mortality rates, and weak health systems. This loss also impacts future policies of these countries, as they are no longer motivated to invest in their medical education systems since the potential returns on investment are diminished. This in turn perpetuates and exacerbates the cycle of human resource shortfalls.

Although the brain drain and brain gain are common occurrences between low income and high-income countries, we are also seeing a new phenomenon of brain circulation. A recent study of Indian students studying in the United States demonstrated a growing number of them returning home to India to pursue their career opportunities after graduation. These opportunities are growing more lucrative alongside India's economic growth and burgeoning technology sector. Other, mainly middle-income countries are also finding ways to entice professionals to return home. One example, is Thailand's Reverse Drain Project, which incentivizes Thai professionals overseas to return home through economic incentives like free housing, salary bonuses, and research grants.

The brain drain, brain gain, and brain circulation raise numerous ethical questions for both individuals and governments. Health professionals in low income countries must make difficult decisions in choosing whether to stay in their home countries, where there is a high need for health professionals, or migrate to high income countries, with better opportunities for advanced training and higher salaries. They should have the autonomy to make this decision on their own. High income countries also face an ethical dilemma- if they encourage health professionals to immigrate, the home countries of these migrants face an even greater shortage of health professionals.

The brain drain is a symptom of an inequitable world. When it occurs, it makes the world even more inequitable. Incentives should be designed to encourage students to stay where the need is the greatest, but allow them the freedom to move if they choose to do so. If a student receive a scholarship or tuition assistance from their home country, they should pay it back with years of service or reimburse their country for the cost if they refuse to do so. Receiving countries also bear a responsibility to pay back poor countries when encouraging migration of health professionals trained abroad.

Access to Medicines & The Role of Pharmaceutical Companies

In the United States alone, we spend around $450 billion on medicines. The pharmaceutical industry is growing at a fast rate, but many criticize their pricing policies and availability of drugs. This section will discuss the research and development of drugs, drug pricing, and the access to drugs. Lifesaving medicines are often unavailable or unaffordable in low income countries and for the poor in high income countries as well. This is clear inequitable and a violation of principles of justice and human rights.

Many pharmaceutical companies argue that their drugs are priced high to account for the high research and development costs in developing these new drugs. A study by the Tufts Center for the Study of Drug Development, estimates that the average costs in the research and development phase of new drugs are estimated to be around $2.9 billion. After the drug is developed, it takes about eight or more years to get it approved by the Food and Drug Administration, and then finally becomes available to the public. Most of these drugs are patent protected for twenty years, which means that other companies are unable to replicate these new drugs on the market. During those twenty years, the patent allows pharmaceutical companies to recover the losses faced during the research and development phase. But there are cases in which some pharmaceutical companies price these new drugs over 5,000% than what it costs to manufacture them, raising the question of whether limits should be placed on the price of life saving drugs.

An example from recent history is the drug Daraprim, produced by Turing Pharmaceuticals. Daraprim is critical in treating a particular opportunistic infection that affects HIV patients. In 2017, Martin Shkreli, then CEO of Turing Pharmaceuticals, hiked the price of Daraprim from $13.50 to $750 per dose. It was estimated that treatment regimens could cost more than $600,000 a year for a patient suffering from toxoplasmosis, a common complication in patients suffering from HIV. This high price of life saving medicine hinders a patient's ability to access treatments and their basic right to a healthy life.

Not only do overpriced drugs pose a problem, but also the lack of medicines in low income countries. One of the reasons for this is because of the low profit margin in these countries. Although there is a high demand for life-saving drugs – few patients in low income countries are able to afford the prices that pharmaceutical companies demand. A study by the WHO shows that over 80% of medications are consumed by only 15% of the world's population, most of whom are in wealthy countries.

This section poses many ethical questions for pharmaceutical companies and governments. Is it ethical for pharmaceutical companies to put expensively priced lifesaving drugs on the market? How do governments encourage the availability of drugs in low income countries without hindering incentives for pharmaceutical companies to invest in drug development? Related to these questions it is important that we keep in mind the core principles of medical ethics – autonomy, beneficence, non-maleficence, and justice. Every person deserves the right a healthy life, no matter their socioeconomic status or geographic location.

- It is important to understand ethical issues pertaining to global health if you plan to participate in an overseas medical experience or support a global health initiative.

- The origins of global health arise out of the exploitation of poor countries during the colonial era.

- Today, there are many positive examples of global health achievements, including smallpox eradication, the global polio eradication initiative, and others.

- Good health and access to health care is considered a human right by the Universal Declaration of Human Rights and many other international and national laws. Health is a key aspect of the global development agenda as framed by the sustainable development goals.

- Achieving good health requires more than just health care and medicines. The social determinants of health describe how income, environment, and behaviors can significantly affect health outcomes. Achieving good health cannot occur in isolation from equality and society at large.

- Over $140 billion in international aid is provided by wealthy countries to poor countries every year. Oftentimes this aid is spent inefficiently or worse, ineffectively. Aid should be participatory and sustainable, making a lasting impact long beyond the specific program being funded.

- Short term medical experiences raise numerous ethical questions related to provision of care by medical trainees or other providers who may be unaware of local norms or customs. These medical "missions" can have distortionary effects on local health systems and often fail to account for follow up care. Short term experiences should only be performed in partnership with local organizations and should focus on supporting local health systems through education and capacity building.

- The brain drain of health professionals from poor to rich countries reflects global inequality and hinders the development of local health systems.

- Lifesaving medications are often unavailable in developing countries. The global pharmaceutical system requires regulation and incentives to ensure that medications are available to all people regardless of their ability to pay or geographic system.

Review Questions

1. The origins of modern global health stem from which historical era?
   a. The global era
   b. The millennial era
   c. The antebellum era
   d. The colonial era

Answer: d. The origins of the modern global health system stem from the colonial era. When European powers were arriving to new, exotic shores they brought with them diseases and strains of bacteria that had never before been encountered. The native populations were exposed to disease such as smallpox, influenza, scarlet fever, and measles, which led to millions of deaths. The European colonizers themselves were also exposed to local diseases. These local diseases would later be referred to as "tropical diseases." Colonizing forces began to bring along their own medical professionals during their colonial conquests in order to control the spread of diseases among their own forces.

2. Which of the following are examples of positive global health initiatives of the modern era?
   a. Smallpox eradication
   b. Global Polio Eradication Initiative
   c. River Blindness eradication efforts
   d. Guinea Worm eradication efforts

Answer: d. All of the above can are positive examples. Smallpox eradication was achieved in 1977. The global polio eradication initiative and efforts to eradicate the infection that causes river blindness are ongoing. The Carter Center for example, has made huge strides leading the global community in the eradication of both guinea worm and river blindness. It works by collaborating with local organizations and training local volunteers to carry out education and disease control interventions.

3. Which document first established health as a fundamental human right?
    a. The Millennium Development Goals
    b. The Universal Declaration of Human Rights
    c. The Sustainable Development Goals
    d. The Alma Ata Declaration

Answer: b. In 1948 the international community codified the rights and freedoms of all individuals through the Universal Declaration of Human Rights. Forty eight countries collaborated on this historic document with the atrocities of World War Two still fresh on the global collective mind. The members of the United Nations agreed to thirty articles protecting human rights. To this day, the Universal Declaration of Human Rights continues to be utilized and implemented through treaties, national constitutions, and laws. Article twenty five of the Universal Declaration of Human Rights, highlights the importance of health as a human right. It states: "Everyone has the right to a standard of living adequate for the health and well-being of himself and of his family, including food, clothing, housing, and medical care and necessary social services, and the right to security in the event of unemployment, sickness, disability, widowhood, old age or other lack of livelihood in circumstances beyond his control." This and other articles of the declaration formed the basis of global development efforts to improve livelihoods in the years that followed.

4. Which document established the global goal of "health for all" with a focus on primary health care?
    a. The Millennium Development Goals
    b. The Universal Declaration of Human Rights
    c. The Sustainable Development Goals
    d. The Alma Ata Declaration

Answer: d. In 1979, the Declaration of Alma Ata was launched at a global primary health care conference, further establishing the importance of accessible primary health care for every person in every country. The Declaration of Alma Ata set a target of health for all by 2000, and tasked the World Health Organization to lead the global community in achieving it. This set the agenda for global public health efforts, highlighting the need to tackle social, economic, and political challenges in order to improve the health of nations and regions.

5. Which document directs the current global development agenda?
    a. The Millennium Development Goals
    b. The Universal Declaration of Human Rights
    c. The Sustainable Development Goals
    d. The Alma Ata Declaration

Answer: c. In 2016, the United Nations updated the global development agenda with the Sustainable Development Goals, or SDGs, setting goals and targets to achieve by 2030. SDG three focuses on ensuring healthy lives and wellbeing for all people of all ages, addressing topics such as maternal and child health, communicable diseases, substance abuse, reproductive health, and universal health care.

6. Which of the following are social determinants of health?
    a. Income
    b. Education
    c. Society
    d. All of the above

Answer: d. All of the above are social determinants of health. According to WHO the three core determinants of health are a person's social and economic environment, physical environment, and their individual characteristics and behaviors. These social determinants of health are all interconnected and affect one another. Social determinants of health touch on health as a human right and one of the core principles of medical ethics – justice. Justice requires that resources are distributed fairly around the world to create societies and environments that are healthy for the people living in them. From birth, these social determinants of health play a critical factor in the quality of life of an individual.

7. Which of the following is a key principle behind successful international aid?
    a. Speed

b. Participation

c. Kickbacks

d. Corruption

Answer: d. Many international organizations come to low income countries with a prearranged plan to eradicate malaria or prevent treat HIV patients. Yet they fail to consult or communicate with people they are serving. Project failure demonstrates the challenge of participatory development. Communities often prioritize different problems while organizations, despite their good intentions, have a different agenda in mind. The challenge for foreign organizations is to involve local people, according to the principle of participation, in project selection, planning, and implementation.

8. What is PEPFAR?
    a. A TB control initiative
    b. A Malaria control initiative
    c. An HIV control initiative
    d. All of the above

Answer: c. The United States President's Emergency Plan for AIDs Relief, better known as PEPFAR, was launched in 2003 as a fifteen billion dollar project to be introduced in around 29 countries. PEPFAR now supports the treatment of over fifty million individuals in in Sub Saharan Africa. Prior to the program, fewer than fifty thousand in the region had access to treatment.

9. Why do medical trainees seek out international medical experiences?
    a. Experience new cultures
    b. Learn about tropical diseases
    c. Develop skills
    d. All of the above

Answer: d. All of the above. Short term medical experiences are when organizations and people come to countries for a few weeks or months to provide service and gain experience working with tropical diseases. This is a particularly common practice for medical students and other trainees. Benefits of participating in these medical experiences include increased knowledge of diverse syndromes and treatments, development of examination skills, and experience with different cultures and religions.

10. What is the "brain drain"?
    a. Transfer of brain tissue samples across borders
    b. Migration from wealthy to poor countries
    c. Migration from poor countries to wealthy countries
    d. All of the above

Answer: c. Brain drain is defined as a migration of highly skilled health professionals from low income to high income countries. On the receiving end are the high-income countries who reap a brain gain from immigration of these highly skilled professionals. They get to enjoy the health and economic benefits of hosting these individuals without having to bear the cost of training them.

Chapter 8: Research Ethics

Ethics plays a significant role in medical research, particularly related to human experimentation. Human subject research can take the form of either observational or interventional research. Medical research most often refers to interventional research methods, such as clinical trials related to new therapies. Clinical trials are used to evaluate the efficacy of drugs, vaccines, or medical devices for future use by the general public. Because of their invasive nature, clinical trials are heavily regulated by many different agencies, agreements, and laws. Those performing research on human subjects are bound by the principles espoused by these international agreements. These include the Declaration of Helsinki, the Nuremberg Code, national laws and regulations, as well as local requirements by institutional or hospital review boards. In the United States, organizations like the Food and Drug Association and the National Institutes of Health provide oversight over this process. There are also recommended good practice documents, such as the European Charter for Researchers, which provide a framework of best practices when working with human subjects.

Informed Consent, Beneficence, and Non-maleficence

Informed consent is likely one of the main issues that come to mind when you think about research ethics. Informed consent directly connects with the principle of autonomy, an individual's right to consent to or refuse any course of treatment - in this case, through a research study. Many of the worst cases of research malpractice in history failed to obtain informed consent from the research subjects. Performing the research either against the subjects' will or without their knowledge. Next, the explicit mandate of non-maleficence, or doing no harm, is an important part of performing research that impacts human subjects. Finally, research involving human subjects is often invasive, requiring individuals to take medications, comply with certain lifestyle changes, and be monitored and probed. Some of these individuals may suffer painful side effects, stress, and other symptoms as a result of the research. For this reason, researchers must consider the costs and benefits of performing the experiment. In other words, the potential benefits of the research must far outweigh the costs to participants. In a way, this is a form of the principle of beneficence, but on a grander scale. During research studies with human subjects, the intent is not only to try to achieve good by developing a new drug, vaccine or medical device/technique that will eventually improve people's lives, but also to minimize the negative effects of the experiments on participants.

Nazi Experiments during World War II

The Nazi experimentation on human subjects during World War II is perhaps one of the most globally recognized abuses of the principles of informed consent and non-maleficence. The Nazis performed painful, often sadistic experiments on many people they considered subhuman, including Jewish people, the Roma, homosexuals, disabled individuals, and political dissidents. Many of their experiments were intended to assist the war effort. These included placing prisoners in pressure chambers to determine safe altitude for ejecting pilots from airplanes, and exposing prisoners to cold temperatures to study hypothermia. The Nazis also worked with pharmaceutical companies and research institutes in Germany to study treatments for malaria and tuberculosis.

These experiments violated a number of important principles in medical ethics: autonomy and informed consent, non-maleficence, and beneficence. The researchers performed experimentation on most, if not all of the subjects against their will. Additionally, the experiments were carried out with little regard for the subjects themselves, but with the ultimate objective of understanding the science. In the Nazi experiments on human subjects, often times the benefits did not outweigh the costs to the research subjects, many of whom perished or suffered severe trauma.

At the end of the war, a series of military tribunals were held in Nuremberg, Germany charging many in the Nazi leadership with war crimes. The Nuremberg trials began with the indictments of twenty three Nazi physicians involved in genocide and unethical experimentation in concentration camps. These physicians were also charged with sterilizing over three million people to eliminate so-called genetic defects from the German gene pool.

Shortly after the trials, the judges used six of the arguments developed by the expert medical advisors for the prosecution to lay out what would eventually become the Nuremberg Code on research ethics. The judges included an additional four points, ultimately outlining ten principles to be applied to medical research involving human subjects. With a focus on informed consent, beneficence, and non-maleficence, these principles are thought to be based on the Hippocratic Oath.

The 10 principles of the Nuremberg Code are as follows:

- Required is the voluntary, well-informed, understanding consent of the human subject in a full legal capacity.
- The experiment should aim at positive results for society that cannot be procured in some other way.
- It should be based on previous knowledge (e.g., an expectation derived from animal experiments) that justifies the experiment.
- The experiment should be set up in a way that avoids unnecessary physical and mental suffering and injuries.
- It should not be conducted when there is any reason to believe that it implies a risk of death or disabling injury.
- The risks of the experiment should be in proportion to (that is, not exceed) the expected humanitarian benefits.
- Preparations and facilities must be provided that adequately protect the subjects against the experiment's risks.
- The staff who conduct or take part in the experiment must be fully trained and scientifically qualified.
- The human subjects must be free to immediately quit the experiment at any point when they feel physically or mentally unable to go on.
- Likewise, the medical staff must stop the experiment at any point when they observe that continuation would be dangerous.

1964 Declaration of Helsinki

Nearly two decades after the Nuremberg Trials, the international community came together to further evaluate the state of ethics related to research. The Declaration of Helsinki is a set of ethics principles developed by the World Medicine Association (WMA) in Helsinki, Finland in 1964. The Declaration of Helsinki represents the first time that the medical community came together to develop standards for human research in an effort to self-regulate. Although it does not have binding power in international law, the Declaration of Helsinki is widely considered one of the most influential documents on human research ethics to this day, influencing countless national and regional laws and regulations governing researching ethics. The document has since been revised multiple times, and focuses on an individual's right to self-determination and informed consent, that the participant's well-being takes precedence over the science, and that ethical considerations come before laws and regulations.

Tuskegee Syphilis Experiments

From the 1930s to the 1970s, the United States Public Health Service began studying a group of over six hundred African American men in collaboration with Tuskegee University. A large proportion of the men were already infected with Syphilis, and the study secretly aimed to determine how and when individuals infected with syphilis should be treated. During the experiments, the men were told they were being treated for "bad blood," a colloquialism referring to several different diseases including syphilis and anemia. The researchers notably did not inform the individuals with syphilis of their condition. Furthermore, even after it was known that penicillin was an effective treatment for syphilis, the men were not appropriately treated, and were even prevented from seeking treatment. This experiment violated the informed consent principle by the doctors' withholding of the true nature of the experiment. It also violated the principles of beneficence and non-maleficence, by not treating the patients or allowing them to seek effective medical treatment. This example of harmful experimentation has resulted in a considerable loss of trust in certain demographic groups that remains today, affecting some individuals' decisions to seek much-needed medical care.

In 1951, Henrietta Lacks was biopsied for a cervical cancer tumor at Johns Hopkins Hospital. During the course of her treatment, samples of her cervix were taken without her permission or knowledge. The samples were given to George Otto Gey, a physician and cancer researcher. While he was studying Lacks' tumor, he noticed that her cells divided at a higher rate than most cells and could be kept alive for longer periods of time. Later that year, Lacks' died in that same hospital from the cancer, which had metastasized throughout her body. Gey sent his lab assistant to harvest more samples from Lacks' body at the autopsy center.

Lack's cells would later come to be known as "immortal cells," capable of dividing many times and allowing researchers to perform extensive experiments on the same line of cells. This added considerable value to controlled experiments by eliminating the additional variable of experimenting on different cells. The cells, known as HeLa cells, are now one of the most widely used cell lines in medical research and have become commercially successful with over 11,000 patents on her cells. HeLa cells have been used in countless experiments around the world, including research on cancer and HIV, and have helped advance medical science.

And yet, many concerns remain over the issue of consent and privacy. Lacks was never asked permission for medical providers to harvest and use her tissue. Moreover, Lacks' cells became a commercial product, patented many times over and sold to medical labs around the world. Meanwhile, Lacks' own family received no compensation and no control over the use of her cells, or the subsequent publication of the DNA sequence from Lacks' cells. Since that time, several lawsuits have addressed privacy and consent in using patient tissues.

Stem Cells

Stem cells are cells that divide and differentiate into specific cell types to repair damaged body tissues and replenish older cells. Stem cells have made bone marrow transplants possible. They have also paved the way for enhanced research techniques, such as knockout mice, in which researchers "knock out" particular genes to study the effects of these genes on disease.

There are two main types of stem cells: adult and embryonic cells. Following fertilization of an embryo, at the early stages of cell division, stem cells are considered totipotent - able to divide and differentiate into any cell in the body, as well as placental cells. Adult stem cells may be induced to become pluripotent - to differentiate into multiple different cell types in the body.

Recent advances in stem cell research have allowed scientists to develop models of certain tissues by chemically inducing stem cells to differentiate into specific cell types. This research has been especially important in the study of brain cell functions in neurological and psychiatric disorders. However, potential ethical concerns have arisen as these models continue to more closely resemble a functioning human brain. At what point could these tissues experience pain and distress, or store and retrieve memories?

Scientists have also begun transplanting human stem cells into animals, creating what are known as chimeras. This procedure has been successfully performed in pigs and mice. Concerns across all of these experiments involve the potential that these tissues - outside of the human body and intermingled within animal models - will develop some form of human sentience. While scientist could carefully craft experimental parameters to avoid creating the conditions for this, the reality is that human conscience is still little understood.

Despite these concerns, some scientist insist that it would be unethical to stop this research. They argue that this may be the only effective way to study brain tissues and brain functionality, without risking harm to living human subjects.

Key Takeaways

- Informed consent directly connects with the principle of autonomy, an individual's right to consent to or refuse any course of treatment - in this case, through a research study.

- The explicit mandate of non-maleficence, or doing no harm, is an important part of performing research that impacts human subjects.

- The potential benefits of the research must far outweigh the costs or risks to participants, and must adhere to the principle of beneficence. During research studies with human subjects, the intent is not only to try to achieve good by developing a new drug, vaccine or medical device/technique that will eventually improve people's lives, but also to minimize the negative effects of the experiments on participants.

- The Nazi experimentation on human subjects during World War II is perhaps one of the most globally recognized abuses of the principles of informed consent and non-maleficence. The Nazis performed painful, often sadistic experiments on many people they considered subhuman, including Jewish people, the Roma, homosexuals, disabled individuals, and political dissidents.

- At the end of the war, a series of military tribunals were held in Nuremberg, Germany charging many in the Nazi leadership with war crimes. Shortly after the trials, the judges used six of the arguments developed by the expert medical advisors for the prosecution to lay out what would eventually become the Nuremberg Code on research ethics. With a focus on informed consent, beneficence, and nonmaleficence, this code is thought to be based on the Hippocratic Oath.

- The Declaration of Helsinki is a set of ethics principles developed by the World Medicine Association (WMA) in Helsinki, Finland in 1964. The Declaration of Helsinki represents the first time that the medical community came together to develop standards for human research in an effort to self-regulate.

- From the 1930s to the 1970s, the United States Public Health Service began studying a group of over six hundred African American men in collaboration with Tuskegee University. A large proportion of the men were already infected with Syphilis, and the study secretly aimed to determine how and when individuals infected with syphilis should be treated. The researchers notably did not inform the individuals with syphilis of their condition. Furthermore, even after it was known that penicillin was an effective treatment for syphilis, the men were not appropriately treated, and were even prevented from seeking treatment.

- In 1951, Henrietta Lacks was biopsied for a cervical cancer tumor at Johns Hopkins Hospital. During the course of her treatment, samples of her cervix were taken without her permission or knowledge. Lack's cells would later come to be known as "immortal cells," capable of dividing many times and allowing researchers to perform extensive experiments on the same line of cells. The cells, known as HeLa cells, are now one of the most widely used cell lines in medical research and have become commercially successful with over 11,000 patents on her cells. Lacks was never asked permission for medical providers to harvest and use her tissue. Moreover, Lacks' cells became a commercial product, patented many times over and sold to medical labs around the world. Lacks' own family received no compensation and no control over the use of her cells, or the subsequent publication of the DNA sequence from Lacks' cells.

1. Which of the following guide research ethics pertaining to human subjects?

   a. Nuremberg Code

   b. Declaration of Helsinki

   c. National Laws

   d. All of the above

Answer: d. Medical research most often refers to interventional research methods, such as clinical trials related to new therapies. Clinical trials are used to evaluate the efficacy of drugs, vaccines, or medical devices for future use by the general public. Because of their invasive nature, clinical trials are heavily regulated by many different agencies, agreements, and laws. Those performing research on human subjects are bound by the principles espoused by these international agreements. These include the Declaration of Helsinki, the Nuremberg Code, national laws and regulations, as well as local requirements by institutional or hospital review boards. In the United States, organizations like the Food and Drug Association and the National Institutes of Health provide oversight over this process. There are also recommended good practice documents, such as the European Charter for Researchers, which provide a framework of best practices when working with human subjects.

2. What is the main issue pertaining to an individual's right to participate or refuse to participate in a study?

   a. Beneficence

   b. Nonmaleficence

   c. Autonomy

   d. Justice

Answer: c. Informed consent is likely one of the main issues that comes to mind when you think about research ethics. Informed consent directly connects with the principle of autonomy, an individual's right to consent to or refuse any course of treatment - in this case, through a research study. Many of the worst cases of research malpractice in history failed to obtain informed consent from the research subjects. Performing the research either against the subjects' will or without their knowledge.

3. Which of the following specific groups were targeted by Nazi Experiments?
    a. Jews
    b. Roma
    c. Homosexuals
    d. All of the above

Answer: d. The Nazi experimentation on human subjects during World War II is perhaps one of the most globally recognized abuses of the principles of informed consent and nonmaleficence. The Nazis performed painful, often sadistic experiments on many people they considered subhuman, including Jewish people, the Roma, homosexuals, disabled individuals, and political dissidents.

4. Where were the trials of Nazi war crimes performed?
    a. Vienna
    b. Nuremberg
    c. Prague
    d. Berlin

Answer: b. At the end of the war, a series of military tribunals were held in Nuremberg, Germany charging many in the Nazi leadership with war crimes. The Nuremberg trials began with the indictments of twenty three Nazi physicians involved in genocide and unethical experimentation in concentration camps. These physicians were also charged with sterilizing over three million people to eliminate so-called genetic defects from the German gene pool.

5. Which of the following documents is considered a basis of the Nuremberg Code
    a. The Helsinki Declaration
    b. The NIH Code of Research Ethics
    c. The Montreal Protocol
    d. The Hippocratic Oath

Answer: d. Shortly after the Nuremberg trials, the judges used six of the arguments developed by the expert medical advisors for the prosecution to lay out what would eventually become the Nuremberg Code on research ethics. The judges included an additional four points, ultimately outlining ten principles to be applied to medical research involving human subjects. With a focus on informed consent, beneficence, and nonmaleficence, these principles are thought to be based on the Hippocratic Oath.

6. Which ethical code was designed in 1964 to govern medical research?
    a. The Nuremberg Code
    b. The Montreal Protocol
    c. The Helsinki Declaration
    d. The FDA Protocol

Answer: c. Nearly two decades after the Nuremberg Trials, the international community came together to further evaluate the state of ethics related to research. The Declaration of Helsinki is a set of ethics principles developed by the World Medicine Association (WMA) in Helsinki, Finland in 1964. The Declaration of Helsinki represents the first time that the medical community came together to develop standards for human research in an effort to self-regulate. Although it does not have binding power in international law, the Declaration of Helsinki is widely considered one of the most influential documents on human research ethics to this day, influencing countless national and regional laws and regulations governing research ethics. The document has since been revised multiple times, and focuses on an individual's right to self-determination and informed consent, that the participant's well-being takes precedence over the science, and that ethical considerations come before laws and regulations.

7. What disease was studied during the Tuskegee experiments?
    a. Syphilis
    b. Chlamydia
    c. Gonorrhea
    d. Diarrhea

Answer: a. From the 1930s to the 1970s, the United States Public Health Service began studying a group of over six hundred African American men in collaboration with Tuskegee University. A large proportion of the men were already infected with Syphilis, and the study secretly aimed to determine how and when individuals infected with syphilis should be treated. During the experiments, the men were told they were being treated for "bad blood," a colloquialism referring to several different diseases including syphilis and anemia. The researchers notably did not inform the individuals with syphilis of their condition. Furthermore, even after it was known that penicillin was an effective treatment for syphilis, the men were not appropriately treated, and were even prevented from seeking treatment.

8. Why are HeLa cells considered valuable?
    a. Cells divide faster and can be kept alive longer
    b. Cells divide slower and can be kept alive longer
    c. Cells mutate faster and can be kept alive longer
    d. Cells do not divide

Answer: a. In 1951, Henrietta Lacks was biopsied for a cervical cancer tumor at Johns Hopkins Hospital. During the course of her treatment, samples of her cervix were taken without her permission or knowledge. The samples were given to George Otto Gey, a physician and cancer researcher. While he was studying Lacks' tumor, he noticed that her cells divided at a higher rate than most cells and could be kept alive for longer periods of time.

9. How many patents are based on HeLa cells?
    a. One
    b. One Hundred
    c. One Thousand
    d. More than Ten Thousand

Answer: d. HeLa cells are known as "immortal cells," capable of dividing many times and allowing researchers to perform extensive experiments on the same line of cells. This added considerable value to controlled experiments by eliminating the additional variable of experimenting on different cells. They are now one of the most widely used cell lines in medical research and have become commercially successful with over 11,000 patents on her cells. HeLa cells have been used in countless experiments around the world, including research on cancer and HIV, and have helped advance medical science.

10. What type of stem cell can be induced to divide and differentiate into any cell type?
    a. Bone Marrow
    b. Cardiac
    c. Embryonic
    d. Liver

Answer: c. There are two main types of stem cells: adult and embryonic cells. Following fertilization of an embryo, at the early stages of cell division, stem cells are considered totipotent - able to divide and differentiate into any cell in the body, as well as placental cells. Adult stem cells may be induced to become pluripotent - to differentiate into multiple different cell types in the body.

Chapter 9: Decision Making in Ethical Dilemmas

In this concluding chapter, we will revisit some of the ethical dilemmas discussed in this course, and present some additional topics in healthcare that are currently subject to intense debate. We will also discuss some strategies when confronted by conflicts of interest and the need for ethical decision-making.

As the previous chapters have shown, doctors are faced with ethical choices every day during their practice of medicine, clinical research, or in their educational roles. Their decisions may be time sensitive, sometimes requiring decisions within hours or minutes. Ethical dilemmas vary in their gravity or impact - is it a life or death situation? Will the patient's quality of life be impacted in some way? And they may be juggling cost control issues imposed by their workplace that could influence their prescribing or lead to denial of care based on a patient's insurance coverage or lack thereof for certain treatments and procedures. Establishing an ethical decision-making framework is important not only for the health providers themselves, but also for transparency and clarity for their patients.

Commonly arising ethical dilemmas include the following: resolving informed consent cases where patients or their family members refuse to consent for medically necessary procedures; interpreting confusing advanced directives; making decisions in end of life situations including cases of medical futility; navigating religious or cultural perspectives of patients; and resolving conflicts related to pregnancy or care for children.

Definition of an Ethical Dilemma

Ethical dilemmas occur when decisions must be made and conflicts of interest arise while balancing differing guidance from the fundamental principles presented earlier in Chapter 1. These principles include:

Autonomy - Has the patient been adequately informed to be able to consent to or refuse the treatment or procedure? Are their choices and values being respected? ;

Justice - Are scarce resource being fairly distributed, are there competing needs? Have all rights and obligations been considered? Does it uphold existing laws?

Beneficence - Will the treatment or procedure ultimately be beneficial for the patient involved? And

Non-maleficence - Do the benefits out-way any adverse risks to the patient?

Ethical dilemmas can also emerge when a doctor's recommendation and the choice of their patient or designated guardian are at odds. Or in situations when a doctor may not share the same moral values as their patient, leading to perceptions of bias. Can a physician decline to follow through with a patient's choice, or refuse to provide care, and what are the limits to conscientious refusal?

End-of-life care for example, which was presented in Chapter 5, is fraught with ethical dilemmas not only for physicians, but for ethicists, lawyers, policy-makers, and family members. Here we will dive into some of decisions doctors make within the last 3 months and last 48 hours of their patients' lives. We will discuss some of the controversies surrounding the idea of futility - at what point does the care that is being provided become futile, or change from doing good according to the beneficence principle to maleficence- to prolonging suffering?

Steps for Effective Decision-Making

Learning to communicate with patients and making fair and ethical decisions are all a part of the physician's profession.

What are some steps for effective decision-making? Physicians must first recognize that they face an ethical dilemma and identify the decision to be made. They must then gather information from the patient, consultants, and colleagues. Alternative choices must be identified and weighed against the information pertaining to the case at hand. The physician and patient, or their representative, must then choose from among the choices and take action.

The most effective strategy is to employ a shared decision-making process, in which the best decision is negotiated in partnership with the patient, responding to their concerns, and preferences.

Ethical framework for Decision-Making

In modern times, two core values have come to dominate the discussion of medical ethics and the key behaviors of doctors: altruism and obligation.

Altruism refers to the fact that a doctor primarily works for the best interests of others, or their patients. Through their behavior, it means that they must work for the benefit of their patients. When patients place their trust and confidence in their physicians to act in their best interest, the doctor then has an obligation, or a fiduciary responsibility to fulfill that trust. We can add to these two core values other generally accepted rules of ethical conduct, namely:

The Golden Rule - referring to reciprocity as described by the classic phrase, do unto others as you would have done unto you.

Impartiality - providing care without any distinction or discrimination, with the added significance of giving priority to those most in need.

The universalizability test- would a provider feel comfortable if all practitioners acted similarly?

Interpersonal justifiability- can physician provide good reasons for their action that their peers would understand and agree with?

The American Medical Association has codified these virtues in their ethical statements outlining the standards of conduct for honorable physicians. These standards state that physicians must be dedicated to providing competent care with compassion, and should uphold high standards of professionalism.

The humanitarian aid organization Doctors without Borders also has guiding principles based on ethical medical practice in relation to global health work. These promote humane treatment free from financial, political, or ideological pressure.

The virtues and principles of conduct discussed in this section provide a moral compass for physicians when faced with difficult decisions from the beginning of life, to the end of life, and everything in-between.

"Rationing" of Limited Resources

Over the last four decades, the state of healthcare in the United States has been characterized by rising costs and debate on how to provide efficient and equitable care to all. In 1980 the US spent approximately eight percent of its GDP on healthcare, which steadily climbed to eighteen percent in 2016. This translated to more resources spent per person on healthcare compared with other wealthy countries. Yet the increase in spending has not translated into better health outcomes or gains in life expectancies.

Some firmly believe that the US healthcare system has been rationed based on income, type of employment, and pre-existing medical conditions. Rationing in purely economic terms is defined as the study of how individuals or society respond to and deal with scarcity. Any limits on the distribution of scarce goods or services is called rationing, whether by pricing or other methods like lotteries and waiting lists.

A few contributing factors can be identified that are driving healthcare costs. These include the cost of new technologies and drugs, the rise of chronic diseases, and high administrative costs. The current employer-financed health insurance system has left many Americans uninsured. In 2014, there were thirty two million uninsured Americans, nine million fewer than the year before, most likely attributable to the implementation of the Affordable Care Act, or ACA. In 2014 only forty nine percent of adult Americans reported being covered by health insurance through their employer. Prohibitive costs have been the main reason Americans give for problems accessing health care.

START Triage

Here is another example of impartial, equitable, and ethical treatment given scarce resources. First responders and doctors that are involved in mass-casualty situations are required to make care decisions quickly and efficiently. They do this by using a method called START triage - which stands for simple triage and rapid treatment. Using this method, victims are quickly classified based on the severity of their injuries. This sometimes means that responders have to purposefully leave some patients behind.

This triage method was developed in 1983 and is currently widely used across the world. First responders that arrive at a mass-casualty scene quickly assess the victims and classify them into 4 categories that are color-coded as red for immediate care, yellow for delayed care, green for minor care, and black for deceased or beyond treatment. The colors represent triage tags, but actual tags do not have to be used if victims can be physically sorted in different areas. The method is primarily used to determine who gets treated and who gets evacuated to a hospital first. A live patient triaged as black will not be transported and will be allowed to die in the field.

START was a significant step forward in dealing with mass casualties due to its emphasis on making a rapid assessment of each patient, determining which of the four categories they should belong to, and visibly identifying them for rescuers who could then begin to treat them in the order identified. In this way, the rescuers would be directed to those patients who had immediate life-threatening injuries and who had the best chance of surviving. It was based on the concept of the golden hour, a concept that if a trauma patient receives advanced care within the first hour of their injury, they have a higher chance of surviving.

In Chapter 6 we first explored the Physician Patient relationship. This section will discuss conscientious refusal by physicians. Can doctors refuse to perform a procedure, for example, if their moral views on it conflict with those of the patient? Can they override a patient's do not resuscitate order if they think their patient has a chance for a meaningful extension of life?

Doctors and other providers may not see eye to eye with decisions made by their patients about their own health or healthcare. Such situations are normal and underlie the American model for informed consent and respect for patient autonomy. When it comes to reproductive rights and the divisive views on whether pregnancy termination or contraception are acceptable, conscientious refusals to perform such procedures have been widespread across the country.

A doctor who employs conscientious refusal may be upholding their personal autonomy and their moral integrity. While conscience is useful in ethical decision-making, it can also lead to professional conflicts of interests. It can lead to a refusal to respect a patient's autonomy, result in adverse outcomes, and erode trust in the doctor patient relationship.

How do we set limits on conscientious refusal? There are four benchmarks against which they can be evaluated. Firstly, we can ask to what degree is the doctor imposing their own beliefs on the patient? Respect for a patient's autonomy means acknowledging their right to decision-making and enabling them to make those decisions for themselves. Providing complete, scientific and accurate information about all options available is prescribed in the oath doctors take.

Secondly, we must evaluate the impact the refusal might have on the well-being of the patient, and particularly the potential for harm. A doctor has a fiduciary duty to act on behalf of the best interests of the patient and protect the patient from harm.

Thirdly, we must evaluate the scientific integrity of the claims for conscientious refusal. Are they based on facts or misinformation? Above all, medicine is committed to scientific evidence and best practice standards across their profession. When claims go against the body of sound evidence, they should not be considered valid.

And finally, the potential for discrimination should be evaluated. Justice is an important concept for doctors and medical ethics - all individuals should be treated fairly and medical care should be provided in a non-discriminatory manner.

Overall, while conscience is important, conscientious refusals should be limited in their use as they can impose religious or moral beliefs on others, may affect a patient's physical or mental health negatively, be based on scientific misinformation, or reinforce racial biases and socioeconomic disparities.

A physician is responsible for providing unbiased and accurate information so their patients can make informed decisions. If their moral conscience causes them to not be able to fulfill that responsibility to the full extent, they must provide their patients with advanced notice. They then have a duty to refer their patients to other providers who can provide the needed services in a timely manner.

End of Life Care

This section will discuss decision making during end of life care. Physicians play a key role in the end of life decision making process, especially in making decisions about initiating a particular course of treatment, withholding medications, or withdrawing life-sustaining devices.

Medical end of life decisions in the last three months of life can include continuation of care at home versus a nursing home, referral to palliative care, withdrawal of treatments, and counseling regarding a do not resuscitate order.

Once a patient's condition progresses to their final days and hours of life, physicians are involved in decisions regarding hospice care, procedures like venous catheters, intubation, urinary catheters, and blood transfusions. All of these interventions may prolong life, but they may not add quality to the patient's final moments.

Ultimately the physician's goal in determining which measures to take in the case of the terminally ill rests on the principle of avoiding unnecessary suffering for the patient.

Studies related to end of life decisions reveal the difficulties physicians face in recognizing a patient's proximity to death and or adequately documenting them in their reports. This may be related to a number of factors, including not wanting to make a mistake, the weight of a terminal diagnosis, and the desire to project a positive attitude for the patient.

As some researchers found while reviewing clinical histories, even when advanced conditions were present, patients were provided with invasive interventions like mechanical ventilations, parenteral nutrition, and transfusions.

Physicians may sometimes be asked to provide assistance to hasten death in the face of a terminal condition. This practice is known as physician assisted suicide and was discussed in chapter 5.

In Oregon, where physicians have been permitted to provide aid and comfort for dying patients for over twenty years, data indicate that one out of every two hundred people consider using the option to actually ingest the lethal drugs that can be prescribed. About half change their minds after getting better symptom management or support for quality of life.

The best decision-making strategy may be to encourage healthy patients to consider writing an advanced directive or living will and designate a surrogate to make healthcare decisions when they cannot.

Advanced directives can take the form of a proxy directive, instructional directive, or both. A proxy directive is when the patient designates a person, or surrogate, to make healthcare decisions on their behalf when they are no longer able to do so. Instructional directives provide written instructions on how a patient would like to be cared for at the end of life, and comes into play when they are no longer able to make the decisions due to incapacity or unable to make their preferences known.

Futile Care

At the end of life for patients with terminal conditions, providing certain types of healthcare is considered a futile exercise or of no medical benefit. In some cases, providing healthcare, or using advanced medical technologies to prolong life, can be considered harmful if associated with pain and complications without any expected benefit.

In cases of disagreement with regard to the care provided in end of life decision making, the autonomy principle should guide the care received. While the right to refuse care by patients is often followed without any caveats, when patients demand care in the face of futility it is difficult for health providers to refuse to provide it.

A recent opinion piece in the New York Times by cardiologist Sandeep Jauhar estimated that there are at least twelve thousand so called futility cases in the United States every year, where patients or their families request invasive care and procedures despite counseling that the care is futile. While rationing and futility are separate ideas, they perhaps should be linked in our technologically advanced system. These cases are associated with significant expenses and use of resources that ultimately may not be useful for the patient, or considered as money well spent.

A large number of such cases are resolved through mediations between physicians and patients' families or mediation by medical ethics teams. But many go unresolved. For most doctors, these cases present a crisis of conscience - how do they obey a central pillar of the profession - to do no harm - when they are forced to provide treatments that prolong suffering?

Generally, disputes such as these are governed by state laws, but these are inconsistent from state-to-state. In Texas, for example, a medical team can withdraw treatment after ten days if a hospital ethics committee agrees that further therapy is futile. But in New York, doctors must continue to provide such treatment indefinitely unless family members agree to withdraw treatment.

Some doctors and healthcare providers advocate the use of the term "allow natural death", which has been adopted in many facilities across the US, to replace "do not resuscitate." This steers the conversation from what will not be delivered to what can and will. Under these circumstances, providers highlight the treatments that they will provide up until the moment of natural death, and then will not attempt CPR or defibrillation or mechanical ventilation to artificially prolong life.

Medical Ethics and the Law

The disputes mentioned in the previous section show how medical ethics often comes in contact with the law, thereby affecting the decision-making process.

Medical ethics have long been influenced and shaped by the legal framework in the US, supported by and consisting of judicial opinions, statutes, and administrative rulings. Each of the fifty states of the US is its own jurisdiction, and the federal government provides its own interpretations. Under the Supremacy Clause of the US Constitution, federal law supersedes state law. Yet not all medical ethics issues are covered and new ones have arisen in which there is no federal law or judicial ruling. Also, judicial opinions that have been made in the past can change over time.

While courts and legislatures put great emphasis on personal autonomy, it's not always the deciding factor. In the case of Schloendorff verses the Society of New York Hospital, Mary E.

Schloendorff was evaluated for a stomach problem. She agreed to an exam with the use of ether anesthesia to find out more about a fibroid tumor. But while she was unconscious from the ether the doctors not only examined her tumor, they removed it. The judge in the case ruled in her favor citing patient autonomy, asserting that she had been assaulted by the procedure since she did not consent to it.

In another famous case, Karen Ann Quinlan entered a persistent vegetative state after suffering respiratory failure, and was kept on life support, which included a mechanical ventilator. Her parents, considering it extraordinary means of prolonging her life that was causing her pain, asked that her ventilator be removed, which her physician and hospital refused. They filed a suit on September 12, 1975 in the New Jersey Superior Court, which ruled in favor of the doctors, calling it a medical decision and not a judicial one. The Quinlans appealed the ruling and the Supreme Court of New Jersey then ruled on their behalf, granting them their wish on March 31, 1976, citing the right to privacy and extending that right to the Quinlans to make the decision on the patient's behalf. Ann Quinlan was removed from the ventilator but a feeding tube was still allowed. She continued to breathe unaided, and later was moved to a nursing home, and passed away almost nine years later due to complications of pneumonia.

The landmark US Supreme Court case in 1990, Cruzan versus the Missouri Department of Health also involved a woman in a persistent vegetative state following a car crash. The legal argument was whether the State of Missouri had the right to require clear evidence from the Cruzan family to remove their daughter from life support. The case was the first right-to-die case argued at the Supreme Court and led to the creation of the advance health directives previously described.

Experimental Drugs and the Placebo

Research scenarios also raise a variety of ethical decision making dilemmas as discussed in chapter 8. Would family members, communities, and healthcare workers accept the randomizing of patient care for scientific research when the risk of death is over 50%, as is the case of Ebola in West Africa? Is it ethical for the drugs to be given in randomized, controlled trials — considered the gold standard in research methodology — since that would require some patients to take placebos? How would you select those patients and would you be obligated to inform them in advance?

These are questions to be raised by the institutional review board that approves research study protocols. These boards are administrative bodies created to protect the rights and welfare of human participants of research studies. They can be established by research institutes, government funding bodies, universities, or individual health facilities. Research studies may need approval from multiple review boards before they can commence. For example, an NIH funded study carried out by a university in a hospital may need separate approval from the NIH, the university, and the hospital in question.

Hospital Ethics Committees

Hospital ethical committees are established by health facilities to deal with ethical concerns raised by any member of the health care team, the patient, or their family. They provide consultations free of charge on a confidential basis as part of a patient's care.

Examples of scenarios evaluated by these committees include times when there is uncertainty around who should make healthcare decisions when a patient is too sick to decide on their own. They can evaluate scenarios when there is conflict between values or religious beliefs and a recommended course of treatment. A common dilemma occurs when there is disagreement around starting, continuing, or ending life sustaining treatments such as breathing tubes or feeding tubes.

Key Takeaways

- Approaches to ethical decision making include the golden rule, the impartiality test, the universalizability test, and interpersonal justifiability test.
- The provision of healthcare is limited by scarce resources, so health systems must devise strategies to provide care in an equitable manner. During mass casualty

scenarios, the START triage protocol helps to maximize the benefit of care to the patients who need it the most.

- Physicians sometimes object to performing requested procedures based on their own belief systems. A doctor who employs conscientious refusal is not only upholding their personal autonomy, but also their moral integrity. While conscience is useful in ethical decision-making, it can also lead to professional conflicts of interests. It can lead to a refusal to respect a patient's autonomy, result in adverse outcomes, and erode trust in the doctor patient relationship.

- Physicians must direct the care of patients in the months and days leading up to the end of their lives. Medical end of life decisions in the last three months of life can include continuation of care at home versus a nursing home, referral to palliative care, withdrawal of treatments, and counseling regarding a do not resuscitate order. Once a patient's condition progresses to their final days and hours of life, physicians are involved in decisions regarding hospice care, procedures like venous catheters, intubation, and urinary catheters, and blood transfusions. All of these interventions may prolong life, but they may not add quality to the patient's final moments.

- At the end of life for patients with terminal conditions, providing certain types of healthcare is considered a futile exercise or of no medical benefit. In some cases, providing healthcare can be considered harmful if associated with pain and complications without any expected benefit. In cases of disagreement with regard to the care provided in end of life decision making, the autonomy principle should guide the care received. While the right to refuse care by patients is often followed without any caveats, when patients demand care in the face of futility it is difficult for health providers to refuse to provide it.

- Medical ethics have long been influenced and shaped by the legal framework in the US, supported by judicial opinions, statutes, and administrative rulings. Each of the fifty states of the US is its own jurisdiction, and the federal government provides its own interpretations. Under the Supremacy Clause of the US Constitution, federal law supersedes state law. Yet not all medical ethics issues are covered and new ones have arisen in which there is no federal law or judicial ruling. Also, judicial opinions can change over time.

- Institutional review boards approve research study protocols and ensure that research is carried out in a humane and ethical manner. These boards are administrative bodies created to protect the rights and welfare of human participants of research studies. They can be established by research institutes, government funding bodies, universities, or individual health facilities

- Hospital ethical committees are established by health facilities to deal with ethical concerns raised by any member of the health care team, the patient, or their family.

Review Questions

1. Which of the following is a challenge associated with ethical decision making in health?
   a. Time sensitivity
   b. Life and death consequences
   c. Differing perspectives
   d. All of the above

Answer: d. As the previous chapters have shown, doctors are faced with ethical choices every day during their practice of medicine, clinical research, or in their educational roles. Their decisions may be time sensitive, sometimes requiring decisions within hours or minutes. Ethical dilemmas vary in their gravity or impact - is it a life or death situation? Will the patient's quality of life be impacted in some way? And they may be juggling cost control issues imposed by their workplace that could influence their prescribing or lead to denial of care based on a patient's insurance coverage or lack thereof for certain treatments and procedures.

2. Under which situation can an ethical dilemma arise?
   a. Conflicting guidance from key ethical principles
   b. Disagreement between doctor and patient
   c. Differing moral values

d. All of the above

Answer: d. Ethical dilemmas can arise from conflicts between key ethical principles (autonomy, beneficence, non maleficence, and justice) and also emerge when a doctor's recommendation and the choice of their patient or designated guardian are at odds. Or in situations when a doctor may not share the same moral values as their patient, leading to perceptions of bias. Can a physician decline to follow through with a patient's choice, or refuse to provide care, and what are the limits to conscientious refusal?

3. What is the first step a physician should take for effective decision making when faced with an ethical dilemma?
   a. Recognize that the decision is an ethical dilemma
   b. Gather information
   c. Counsel the patient
   d. Consult an ethics committee

Answer: a. Physicians must first recognize that they face an ethical dilemma and identify the decision to be made. They must then gather information from the patient, consultants, and colleagues. Alternative choices be identified and weighed against the information pertaining to the case at hand. The physician and patient, or their representative, must then choose from among the choices and take action.

4. Which of the following are accepted rules for ethical conduct for physicians?
   a. Altruism
   b. Obligation
   c. The Golden Rule
   d. All of the above

Answer: d. In modern times, two core values have come to dominate the discussion of medical ethics and the key behaviors of doctors: altruism and obligation. Altruism refers to the fact that a doctor primarily works for the best interests of others, or their patients. Through their behavior, it means that they must work for the benefit of their patients. When patients place their trust and confidence in their physicians to act in their best interest, the doctor has a fiduciary responsibility, or obligation to fulfill that trust. The

Golden Rule refers to reciprocity as described by the classic phrase, do unto others as you would have done unto you.

5. Which of the following is a definition of the impartiality test?
    a. Reciprocity
    b. Providing good reasons
    c. Care without prejudice or discrimination
    d. Provider would be comfortable if all physicians acted the same

Answer: c. The golden rule refers to reciprocity as described by the classic phrase, do unto others as you would have done unto you. The impartiality tests means that doctors provide care without any distinction or discrimination, with the added significance of giving priority to those most in need. The universalizability test asks if a provider would feel comfortable if all practitioners acted similarly. The interpersonal justifiability test asks if a physician can provide good reasons for their action that their peers would understand and agree with.

6. Which of the following is a definition of the interpersonal justifiability test?
    a. Reciprocity
    b. Providing good reasons
    c. Care without prejudice or discrimination
    d. Provider would be comfortable if all physicians acted the same

Answer: b. The golden rule refers to reciprocity as described by the classic phrase, do unto others as you would have done unto you. The impartiality tests means that doctors provide care without any distinction or discrimination, with the added significance of giving priority to those most in need. The universalizability test asks if a provider would feel comfortable if all practitioners acted similarly. The interpersonal justifiability test asks if a physician can provide good reasons for their action that their peers would understand and agree with.

7. What is an example of ethical rationing?
    a. Refusing care to homeless patients

b. START triage during mass casualty incidents

c. Selling generic medications to uninsured patients

d. All of the above

Answer: b. First responders and doctors that are involved in mass-casualty situations deal with ethical dilemmas and are required to make care decisions quickly and efficiently. They do this by using a method called START triage - which stands for simple triage and rapid treatment (START). Using this method, victims are quickly classified based on the severity of their injuries. This sometimes means that they have to purposefully leave some behind. This triage method was developed in 1983 and is currently widely used across the US. First responders that arrive at a mass-casualty scene quickly assess the victims and classify them into 4 categories that are color-coded as red for immediate care, yellow for delayed care, green for minor care, and black for deceased or beyond treatment. The colors represent triage tags, but actual tags do not have to be used if victims can be physically sorted in different areas. The method is primarily used to determine who gets treated and who gets evacuated to a hospital first. A live patient triaged as black will not be transported and will be allowed to die in the field.

8. Which of the following refers to the practice of doctors refusing to provide care that they morally object to?

a. Conscientious refusal

b. Refusal of care

c. Scofflaw

d. Ethics committee review

Answer: a. Doctors and other providers may not see eye to eye with decisions made by their patients about their own health or healthcare. Such situations are normal and underlie the American model for informed consent and respect for patient autonomy. When it comes to reproductive rights and the divisive views on whether pregnancy termination or contraception are acceptable, conscientious refusals to perform such procedures have been widespread across the country. A doctor who employs conscientious refusal is not only upholding their personal autonomy, but also their moral integrity. While conscience is useful in ethical decision-making, it can also lead to professional conflicts of interests. It can lead to a refusal to respect a patient's autonomy, resulting in adverse outcomes, and erode trust in the doctor patient relationship.

9. What is the definition of futile care?
    a. Medical care that hastens death
    b. Medical care that prolongs life
    c. Medical care that provides no medical benefit
    d. All of the above

Answer: c. At the end of life for patients with terminal conditions, providing certain types of healthcare is considered a futile exercise or of no medical benefit. In some cases, providing healthcare can be considered harmful if associated with pain and complications without any expected benefit. In cases of disagreement with regard to the care provided in end of life decision making, the autonomy principle should guide the care received. While the right to refuse care by patients is often followed without any caveats, when patients demand care in the face of futility it is difficult for health providers to refuse to provide it.

10. What hospital board can help when there is a disagreement about the course of treatment needed in difficult situations?
    a. Institutional review board
    b. Hospital ethics committee
    c. Legal department
    d. Office of the hospital CEO

Answer: b. Hospital ethical committees are established by health facilities to deal with ethical concerns raised by any member of the health care team, the patient, or their family. They provide consultations free of charge on a confidential basis as part of a patient's care. Examples of scenarios evaluated by these committees include times when there is uncertainty around who should make healthcare decisions when a patient is too sick to decide on their own. They can evaluate scenarios when there is conflict between values or religious beliefs and a recommended course of treatment. A common dilemma occurs when there is disagreement around starting, continuing, or ending life sustaining treatments such as breathing tubes or feeding tubes

Summary:

This course reviewed medical ethics and included a discussion of many of the unique aspects of the practice of medicine. These included the physician's duty to do good, and sometimes more importantly, to do no harm. Physicians are responsible for ensuring health at the beginning of life, and its end, and throughout the challenging moments in between. They must adhere to an ethical code, and they are held to a high moral standard by society- reflected in the laws and procedures around medical credentialing and licensure.

Chapter 1 provided an overview of medical ethics summarizing the core values of the field which include respect for patient autonomy, beneficence, or doing good for patients, non-maleficence, or not doing harm to patients, and justice. The chapter then reviewed three different philosophical approaches to ethical thinking including utilitarianism, deontology, and virtue ethics. These approaches stem from the philosophical teachings of Jeremy Bentham, John Stuart Mills, Immanuel Kant, and Aristotle, among others.

Chapter 2 discussed the issue of patient competence and decision making capacity, which is linked to the core value of respecting patient autonomy. This chapter discussed situations where patients may not have the ability to make decisions for themselves. The issues of informed consent, competence, and capacity were reviewed here. The special cases of what to do when treating children, people with mental illness, or intoxicated patients were also explored.

Chapter 3 highlighted the importance of patient confidentiality and appropriate use of medical records, an issue that has become particularly important following the digital health revolutions of recent decades. This chapter paid particular attention to exceptions to the confidentiality rule, including reportable conditions and moments where there is a concern for imminent harm.

Chapter 4 discussed one of the most controversial topics in medical ethics, covering issues related to reproductive health. The issue of abortion, for example, has become synonymous with medical ethics over recent decades. The issue becomes more complicated as technology related to fetal imaging and neonatal care continues to advance. Other topics included in this chapter were maternal fetal conflict, sterilization, and the donation of sperm and eggs.

Chapter 5 presented ethical dilemmas associated with end of life care, which have grown more complicated alongside the advancement of medical science and technology. Physicians today have the ability to prolong human life like never before, but this forces the question- should they? Included in this chapter were discussions on advanced directives, withdrawal of treatment, medical futility, and physician assisted suicide.

Chapter 6 covered the physician patient relationship. The chapter defined when the relationship begins and highlighted unique features of this relationship. These features included confidentiality, shared decision making, and the so called fiduciary relationship. It also discussed conflicts of interest, impaired physicians, inappropriate relationships between health providers and their patients, gifts from patients, and disclosure of medical errors.

Chapter 7 reviewed ethical issues in global health. This chapter covered dilemmas faced by Western health providers going to low resource settings to provide care. It also discussed specific ethical issues around global health challenges like HIV/AIDS.

Chapter 8 discussed ethics in medical research, including informed consent of human subjects and modern research dilemmas including the issue of stem cell research.

Chapter 9 concluded this course on medical ethics by providing a decision making framework to address ethical dilemmas. The utilization of review boards and ethics committees were discussed as strategies to take action in the context of ethical conflict.

Review questions:

1. Which of the following is a core principle of medical ethics?

    a. Freedom

    b. Discipline

    c. Utilitarianism

    d. Beneficence

Answer: d. The principle of beneficence states that physicians should only take actions that are beneficial for their patients, or promote well-being and improved health.

2. Which philosopher is commonly associated with virtue ethics?

    a. Jeremy Bentham

    b. Aristotle

    c. Plato

    d. John Locke

Answer: C. Socrates and Plato are usually associated with virtue ethics. This approach relies on character traits and core beliefs, referred to as virtues. These virtues include honesty, humility, generosity, and courage.

3. Which Latin phrase is associated with the definition of nonmaleficence?

    a. *Primum non nocere*

    b. *Auribus teneo lupum*

    c. *Carpe noctum*

    d. *Castigat ridendeo mores*

Answer: a. Nonmaleficence states that physicians should not take any actions that cause harm to their patients. This principle is often summarized by the Latin phrase *primum non nocere*, or first do no harm.

4. Under which of the following scenarios would it generally be permissible to overrule a patient's autonomy while providing medical care?

    a. Dementia

b. Intoxication

c. Psychiatric illness

d. All of the above

Answer: d. Autonomy is the core value behind the concepts of informed consent and shared decision making on medical treatment options. A patient's autonomy, or their personal decision to pursue or refuse treatment, can only be overruled in situations when their capacity is impaired. These include intoxication, psychiatric illness, and dementia.

5. Informed consent in research is an example of which core principle of medical ethics?

   a. Freedom

   b. Autonomy

   c. Utilitarianism

   d. Courage

Answer: b. Autonomy refers to a person's right to consent to and select their desired treatment or participation in any research protocol.

6. Which of the following is a common reason for a minor to be declared "emancipated"?

   a. Patient is highly intelligent

   b. Patient is married

   c. Patient has a full time job

   d. All of the above

Answer: b. "Emancipated" minors are granted their status by a court order, by getting married, or by joining the military. Emancipated minors are considered independent from parental control, and can therefore make healthcare decisions for themselves. Specific laws related to the ability of minors to consent for certain types of treatment and to emancipated minors vary state to state.

7. In certain states, a physician can provide treatment to a minor without parental or legal guardian consent in which of the following circumstances?

a. Patient requests confidentiality

b. Patient is a distant relative

c. Patient has an STD

d. All of the above

Answer: c. In some states, minors may consent for themselves for treatment of sexually transmitted diseases or for health care related to birth control or an active pregnancy.

8. In a case of severe mental illness, under which scenario can a patient be transferred to a psychiatric facility against their will?

   a. Family member request

   b. Imminent threat to others

   c. Medication non-compliance

   d. Disorganized thoughts

Answer: b. While specific laws vary from state to state, most concur that when patients are at imminent risk of self-harm or harm to others they can be transferred to a psychiatric facility against their will. This process is known as involuntary, or civil, commitment.

9. Under which of the following scenarios can a physician use chemical or physical restraints on an uncooperative patient?

   a. Patient disagrees with care plan

   b. Altered mental status from medical illness

   c. Patient refuses to pay for services

   d. All of the above

Answer: b. When patients demonstrate an acute alteration in their mental status associated with a medical illness or intoxication, they are not considered to be competent and able to refuse care. This conclusion is based on the assumption that, were they not confused from their illness or intoxication, they would consent to the treatments being offered.

10. Which of the following statements is correct regarding chemical and physical restraints?

   a. Physical restraints are always preferable to chemical restraints

b. When chemical restraints are used, the maximum dose should be administered

c. When restraints are used, the patient should be reevaluated frequently so as to discontinue the restraints as soon as possible

d. Physical and chemical restraints should be continued for the entire length of the patient's care regardless of the patient's condition

Answer: c. When restraints are used, the patient should be reevaluated frequently so as to discontinue the restraints as soon as possible

11. Which of the following is part of the definition of patient decision making capacity?

   a. Autonomy
   b. Wealth
   c. Reasoning
   d. Legal authority

Answer: c. Decision making capacity evaluation is often summarized by the phrase: understanding, appreciation, reasoning, and ability to express a choice.

12. Which of the following cases represents a breach in patient confidentiality?

   a. Transmitting medical records to another physician with written permission from the patient
   b. Discussing the patient's medical condition with a consulting physician
   c. Discussing the patient's medical condition with another health provider while in a crowded hospital elevator or cafeteria
   d. All of the Above

Answer: c. In practice, adhering to patient confidentiality standards requires vigilance against breaches in patient privacy. Physicians should tell the patient when their information needs to be disclosed for clinical care purposes. Conversations in the hospital cafeteria or in building elevators where others may overhear details are inappropriate.

13. Which of the following is a potential scenario when patient confidentiality may be breached (depending on the legal jurisdiction)?

a. Gunshot or Stab wound report to the police

b. Suspected child abuse

c. Impaired driver report to the department of motor vehicles

d. All of the above

Answer: d. As a general rule, if maintaining patient confidentiality could cause an individual or group harm, then in that case disclosing the information may be allowable. The American Medical Association code on confidentiality concurs with this approach, allowing a breach of confidentiality only in the case of a threat of self-harm or harm to others or when there is a legal requirement to do so. Gunshot and stab wounds are often required to be reported to the police in the interest of public safety and to aid in criminal investigations. Suspected child abuse must be reported to the authorities. Impaired drivers must be reported in order to prevent them from driving and causing accidents.

14. Which of the following scenarios are suspicious for child abuse and should be reported to child welfare authorities?

a. Sprained ankle in 11 year old while playing soccer

b. Multiple old injuries at various stages of healing in an 8 year old who fell down the stairs.

c. Finger crush injury in 8 year old whose hand was caught in the car door

d. All of the above

Answer: b. Cases of child abuse are another example where confidentiality must be breached. In a circumstance where a medical provider suspects abuse, or when the child reports abuse to the provider, the provider is obligated to report the case to the police or other child welfare authority. This scenario often arises with the injuries of a child do not match the history of the event provided by the child or family member. Concerning findings on physical examination may also arouse suspicion, including spiral bone fractures, retinal hemorrhages, and multiple old injuries at various stages of healing.

15. Which of the following diseases is a reportable or notifiable disease?

a. Tuberculosis

b. Pneumonia

c. Respiratory Syncytial Virus

d. Coronavirus

Answer: a. Reportable conditions include highly contagious diseases, vaccine preventable diseases, and diseases that can be associated with bioterrorism. These include measles, meningitis, rabies, anthrax, botulism, chlamydia, gonorrhea, syphilis, tetanus and tuberculosis, to name a few.

16. Which of the following is considered protected health information or PHI?

    a. Laboratory Results

    b. Digital x-ray images

    c. Diagnosis billing code

    d. Patient date of birth

Answer: d. PHI includes any information that can be used to link a medical record to an individual. While the medical record includes health conditions and treatments, patient identifiers under this framework include a patient's name, date of birth, social security number, medical record number, address, email, and photograph.

17. Prior to the advent of intensive care medicine in the 1950's and 1960's, what percentage of people in the United States died at home?

    a. 30%

    b. 50%

    c. 70%

    d. 80%

Answer: c. Prior to the advent of intensive care facilities in hospitals in the 1950s and 60's, the majority of Americans died at home and only about one third died in hospital facilities. Today, the ratio has reversed with only 20% dying at home, and 80% dying in hospitals and nursing homes.

18. Today, what percentage of people in the United States die at home?

    a. 20%

    b. 40%

c. 60%

d. 70%

Answer: a. Prior to the advent of intensive care facilities in hospitals in the 1950s and 60's, the majority of Americans died at home and only about one third died in hospital facilities. Today, the ratio has reversed with only 20% dying at home, and 80% dying in hospitals and nursing homes.

19. Which of the following is a definition of an advanced directive?

   a. A document which names a person able to make decisions for the patient if they are unable to do so

   b. A legal document specifying what actions a patient would like their health providers to take in different situations

   c. A medical order written by the physician that preempts resuscitation if the patient stops breathing or if their heart stops beating

   d. All of the above

Answer: b. An advanced directive is a legal document specifying what actions a patient would like their health providers to take in different situations.

20. What is the legal definition of medical futility?

   a. A terminal illness at any stage

   b. A terminal illness at the final stage

   c. A severe life threatening medical condition or injury

   d. There is no legal definition of medical futility

Answer: d. Withdrawal of treatment can be performed in cases where continuation of these treatments would be considered medically futile. This determination should be made in cooperation with the entire medical care team and the patient's family, as there is no strict legal or medical definition of futility.

21. In what state of the United States is physician assisted suicide legal?

   a. Alabama

   b. Florida

    c. Oregon

    d. Virginia

Answer: c. Oregon is currently the only state in the United States that allows physician assisted suicide. Since the implementation of the state's death with dignity act in 1997, physicians have been permitted to prescribe a lethal dose of a medication to patients with a terminal illness. The illness must have progressed to a stage where the patient has less than six months to live, and a second physician must review the case before the medication is prescribed.

22. What is the definition of physician assisted suicide?

    a. A physician administers a lethal dose of a medication

    b. A physician prescribes a lethal dose of a medication

    c. A physician advises a patient to end their life

    d. All of the above

Answer: b. Physician assisted suicide is defined as a physician providing medications for a patient to end their own life. This could take the form of a prescription for a large dose of morphine or other sedative that the patient would ingest or inject themselves. This definition is in contrast to euthanasia, where a physician would not only prescribe the medication but also administer it.

23. Opponents of legal abortion are usually referred to as what movement?

    a. Pro Abortion

    b. Pro Life

    c. Pro Choice

    d. Anti-Regulation

Answer: b. Those who are against abortion fall into the "pro-life" camp, whereas those who are for women having the right to choose are called, appropriately, "pro-choice." For doctors with this viewpoint, performing an abortion requires the termination of the life of a fetus. Being pro-life hinges on the principle of non-maleficence, or not doing harm to patients, if one looks at the issue from the perspective of the fetus.

24. During the years when abortion was illegal, certain states permitted the practice under exceptional circumstances. These exceptions included which of the following?

   a. Patient preference

   b. Court Order

   c. Danger to the mother

   d. All of the above

Answer: c. During the years when abortion was illegal, some states outlined exceptional circumstances that allowed for the practice to be performed. These circumstances included pregnancy as a result of rape or incest and also when the mother's life was in danger. In this latter case, it was agreed in these locations that the ideal of beneficence to the mother outweighed the non-maleficence to the fetus.

25. Who was the founder of the American Birth Control League?

   a. Susan B Anthony

   b. Margaret Sanger

   c. Ruth Bader Ginsberg

   d. All of the above

Answer: b. The American Birth Control League or ABCL was an organization dedicated to pushing for the creation and promotion of birth control clinics. Its founder, Margaret Sanger, believed that women had the right to control their own fertility, and this included access to abortion. In 1942, the ABCL went on to become the Planned Parenthood Federation of America.

26. Who was the woman identified as Jane Roe in the Supreme Court case Roe v Wade?

   a. Margaret Sanger

   b. Henrietta Wade

   c. Norma McCorvey

   d. Ruth Jones

Answer: c. A Texan woman named Norma McCorvey challenged the abortion law and was referred to in court documents as Jane Roe. McCorvey was pregnant with her third child in

1969. She decided to go against the advice of her friends to lie and claim that she was raped. Instead, she chose to petition for a legal abortion in Texas.

27. Who was "Wade" in the Supreme Court case Roe v Wade?
    a. Henry Wade
    b. Henrietta Wade
    c. Norma McCorvey
    d. Ruth Jones

Answer: c. A Texan woman named Norma McCorvey challenged the abortion law and was referred to in court documents as Jane Roe. McCorvey was pregnant with her third child in 1969. She decided to go against the advice of her friends to lie and claim that she was raped. Instead, she chose to petition for a legal abortion in Texas. In court she faced off against Henry Wade, who was the District Attorney of Dallas County at the time.

28. In the court case *In re Fetus Brown*, what medical procedure did the pregnant woman refuse on religious grounds?
    a. Amniocentesis
    b. Stem cell therapy
    c. Blood donation
    d. Blood transfusion

Answer: d. *In re Fetus Brown* dealt with the issue of maternal religious beliefs. The case occurred when a pregnant woman refused a potentially lifesaving blood transfusion due to a religious objection to the practice.

29. What country undertook a national forced sterilization campaign during its "emergency" period in the late 1970's?
    a. China
    b. India
    c. Pakistan
    d. Indonesia

Answer: b. In 1976, the emergency government regime decided that it needed to take more drastic steps to curb India's rapidly growing population problem. The government decided to put in some very unpopular policies that included compulsory sterilization. Not only did these take away patient autonomy, they also took place in "sterilization camps" that focused on speed and not on safety, resulting in numerous post-procedural complications. The harm done to patients – whether for a doctor's personal gain or otherwise – was a clear violation of the ethical principle of non-maleficence.

30. What are the common critiques against government sponsored sterilization campaigns?
    a. They target the poor
    b. They target the uneducated
    c. They target marginalized social groups
    d. All of the above

Answer: d. Eugenics refers to facilitating and allowing reproduction amongst only the most fit and desirable in society with the intention of creating a better society overall. Government sponsored sterilization programs are often offshoots of this type of thinking and remove the rights of marginalized individuals to be able to have offspring.

31. In the classic ethical thought experiment known as the "trolley dilemma," you are the driver of a trolley car whose brakes have failed. Ahead of you on the track are five individuals who will be struck and killed if you do nothing. You can switch the car to an adjacent track, but that will mean that your action will lead to the death of one person standing on that track. According to the theory of utilitarianism, what action should be taken?
    a. No action
    b. Jump off the trolley
    c. Switch the trolley to the adjacent track
    d. Accelerate the speed of the trolley

Answer: c. According to utilitarian thinking, the driver should switch tracks, killing the individual on track two. Instead of killing five people, the trolley will have then only killed one which is a better outcome in terms of maximizing benefit. Of course, the analysis gets more complicated when additional factors are added in to the scenario. What if the one person on the adjacent track is a child and the five people on track one are elderly? What if the one person on track two is a loved one or relative?

32. In the classic ethical thought experiment known as the "trolley dilemma," you are the driver of a trolley car whose brakes have failed. Ahead of you on the track are five individuals who will be struck and killed if you do nothing. You can switch the car to an adjacent track, but that will mean that your action will lead to the death of one person standing on that track. According to the theory of deontology, what action should be taken?
    a. No action
    b. Jump off the trolley
    c. Switch the trolley to the adjacent track
    d. Accelerate the speed of the trolley

Answer: a. Revisiting the classic runaway trolley problem, deontology provides a different new perspective. According to deontology, it would never be acceptable to take an action that would cause harm. So switching to track number two would be considered unethical since it would lead to a death. Here, the fact that the trolley driver takes an action that causes the death on track number two is important. It is differentiated from the driver taking no action and letting natural events take their course as the trolley collides with the five people on track number one.

33. Which of the following is a potential complication of egg donation?
    a. Menopause like symptoms
    b. Ovarian Torsion
    c. Abdominal swelling
    d. All of the above

Answer: d. It is not as easy to extract an egg as it is to get donor sperm for obvious biological reasons. Female egg donors must first undergo treatment with a hormonal medication to hyperstimulate their ovaries into producing several eggs. Side effects of these medications include allergic reactions, menopause like symptoms, and abdominal swelling. The ovarian stimulation can rarely cause a condition known as ovarian torsion, which can lead to permanent loss of ovarian function. Donors must then undergo a surgical procedure to extract the eggs from their bodies. One study estimated the rate of complications following this surgical procedure to be around two percent. Egg donors may spend over sixty hours of their time through this process in addition to the risks they face taking the medications and undergoing the surgical procedure itself.

34. Which of the following is a potential complication of sperm donation?
    a. Menopause like symptoms
    b. Testicular Torsion
    c. Abdominal swelling
    d. None of the above

Answer: d. Sperm donation is safe for the donor and is not associated with any potential complications.

35. In which of the following countries is euthanasia legally permitted?
    a. The USA
    b. The Netherlands
    c. Canada
    d. Ireland

Answer: b. The definition of physician assisted suicide is in contrast to euthanasia, where a physician would not only prescribe the medication but also administer it. Euthanasia is currently only legally permitted in Belgium, the Netherlands, Columbia, and Luxemburg.

36. What is "brain circulation"?
    a. Transfer of brain tissue samples across borders
    b. Migration from wealthy to poor countries
    c. Migration from poor countries to wealthy countries
    d. Balanced migration between poor and wealthy countries

Answer: d. Balanced migration. Circulation involves an equal number of professionals migrating between low income and high-income countries and back again. In recent years many low and middle-income countries are also finding ways to entice professionals to return home. One example, is Thailand's Reverse Drain Project, which incentivizes Thai professionals overseas to return home through economic incentives like free housing, salary bonuses, and research grants.

37. Which medication saw a price increase of over 5,000% in 2017?
    a. Carbapenem
    b. Daraprim
    c. Zosyn
    d. Amoxicillin

Answer: d. The drug Daraprim, produced by Turing Pharmaceuticals, is critical in treating a particular opportunistic infection that affects HIV patients. In 2017, Martin Shkreli, then CEO of Turing Pharmaceuticals, hiked the price of Daraprim from $13.50 to $750 per dose. It was estimated that treatment regimens could cost more than $600,000 a year for a patient suffering from toxoplasmosis, a common complication in patients suffering from HIV. This high price of life saving medicine hinders a patient's ability to access treatments and their basic right to a healthy life.

38. Which of the following concerns were raised at the time PEPFAR was launched?
    a. Not enough health workers to implement plan
    b. Not enough infrastructure
    c. Africans can't tell time well enough to follow a complex treatment regimen
    d. All of the above

Answer: d. All of the above. USAID administrator Andrew Natsios stated that antiretroviral therapy in Africa would be ineffective since the region lacked trained doctors and adequate infrastructure. He went further by asserting that Africans could not follow a complicated treatment regimen due to their inability to tell time.

39. Which of the following are social determinants of health?

a. Physical environment

b. Blood pressure

c. Diabetes

d. HIV status

Answer: d. According to WHO the three core determinants of health are a person's social and economic environment, physical environment, and their individual characteristics and behaviors. These social determinants of health are all interconnected and affect one another. Social determinants of health touch on health as a human right and one of the core principles of medical ethics – justice. Justice requires that resources are distributed fairly around the world to create societies and environments that are healthy for the people living in them. From birth, these social determinants of health play a critical factor in the quality of life of an individual.

40. How many of the millennium development goals specifically focus on health?

a. None

b. One

c. Four

d. Eight

Answer: c. The Millennium Development Goals set social welfare targets between the year 2000 and 2015. Four of the eight total MDGs specifically focused on health including MDG 1 on poverty and hunger, 4 on child mortality, 5 on maternal health, and 6 on HIV/AIDS and other diseases.

41. How many of the sustainable development goals specifically focus on health?

a. None

b. One

c. Four

d. Eight

Answer: b. In 2016, the United Nations updated the global development agenda with the Sustainable Development Goals, or SDGs, setting goals and targets to achieve by 2030. SDG three focuses on ensuring healthy lives and wellbeing for all people of all ages, addressing topics such as maternal and child health, communicable diseases, substance abuse, reproductive health, and universal health care.

42. Which document directed the global development agenda between 2000 and 2015?
    a. The Millennium Development Goals
    b. The Universal Declaration of Human Rights
    c. The Sustainable Development Goals
    d. The Alma Ata Declaration

Answer: a. The Millennium Development Goals set social welfare targets between the year 2000 and 2015. Four of the eight total MDGs specifically focused on health.

43. Which of the following are examples of positive global health initiatives of the modern era?
    a. Use of covert intelligence operatives as vaccine workers
    b. Guinea Worm eradication efforts
    c. Building hospitals to gather intelligence on local communities
    d. Reductions in the US government international assistance budget

Answer: b. Smallpox eradication was achieved in 1977. The global polio eradication initiative and efforts to eradicate the infection that causes river blindness are ongoing. The Carter Center for example, has made huge strides leading the global community in the eradication of both guinea worm and river blindness. It works by collaborating with local organizations and training local volunteers to carry out education and disease control interventions.

44. The origins of modern global health stem from which historical era?
    a. The colonial era
    b. The post World War II era
    c. The Vietnam war era
    d. The Age of Discovery

Answer: a. The origins of the modern global health system stem from the colonial era. When European powers were arriving to new, exotic shores they brought with them diseases and strains of bacteria that had never before been encountered. The native populations were exposed to disease such as smallpox, influenza, scarlet fever, and measles, which led to millions of deaths. The European colonizers themselves were also exposed to local diseases. These local diseases would later be referred to as "tropical diseases." Colonizing forces began to bring along their own medical professionals during their colonial conquests in order to control the spread of diseases among their own forces.

45. In what situation may a doctor refuse a doctor patient relationship?
    a. Emergency physician who sees a patient in the emergency room
    b. Specialist receives a consultation request when not on duty
    c. Physician refuses to treat patients of a certain ethnicity
    d. All of the above

Answer: b. Doctors may under certain circumstances (e.g. while not on duty) refuse to initiate a doctor patient relationship. The right to refuse care does not apply to doctors working in an emergency room, who must treat all potential patients. It is also not permitted to refuse treatment based on a personal characteristic of the patient as that would be defined as discrimination.

46. According to the fiduciary relationship, the role does the patient play?
    a. Beneficiary
    b. Responsible party
    c. Executor
    d. All of the above

Answer: a. The definition of the fiduciary concept and the example of the fiduciary rule fit well with this discussion on the doctor patient relationship. Here, the physician is the responsible party and the patient is the beneficiary. There is clearly an inequality of power between physicians and their patients, since physicians alone have the medical knowledge that can address a patient's health care needs. They therefore have both a legal and ethical duty according to the definition of a fiduciary relationship.

47. Which of the following is a conflict of interest?

a. Physician receives cash bonuses from colleagues for referrals for specialty care
b. Physician runs their own radiology center and directs their patients there for x-rays
c. Physician receives cash bonuses from the pharmaceutical industry to prescribe certain medications
d. All of the above

Answer: d. A conflict of interest is defined as an opportunity for a person to make personal profit from decisions they are making in their official capacity or profession. Examples from the field of medicine include a physician selling medications or products that they also recommend and prescribe. Even if the medication or product is effective, the obvious conflict of interest may damage the doctor patient relationship if the patient suspects that the doctor is prescribing the treatment to reap personal gain. Similarly, if the physicians receives a kickback or incentive when they prescribe certain medications, a conflict of interest is present. Are they prescribing the medications because it is the best course of treatment for their patients? Or are they doing so in order to receive their commission.

48. Which of the following can cause physician impairment?
a. Alcohol abuse
b. Cocaine abuse
c. Dementia
d. All of the above

Answer: d. Physicians as a group suffer from the same challenges faced by the general population including alcohol and drug abuse, psychiatric illness, and dementia. Alcohol abuse is the most common cause of physician impairment. An estimated eight to twelve percent of physicians will suffer from some form of substance abuse during the course of their careers. Physicians working in the specialties of emergency medicine and anesthesiology are considered to have the highest risk of substance abuse compared with others. Impaired physicians place their patients at risk of medical errors and inappropriate care every day they continue to practice.

49. What characteristics of patient gifts to providers are concerning?

    a. Intimate or romantic oriented gifts

    b. Lavish gift with expectation of special treatment

    c. Cash gift in exchange for prescription refill

    d. All of the above

Answer: d. Most physicians choose the conditional acceptance of gifts. When evaluating an individual gift, they can consider the motivation of the patient in giving it. Is the patient trying to secure preferential treatment? Is the gift itself an inappropriate item indicating romance or other intimacy? Is the gift extravagant? Physicians can also consider the timing of the gift. A gift given in late December for example, may be appropriate and in line with cultural norms of seasonal gift giving.

50. Under which circumstance might a doctor patient relationship be acceptable?

    a. Rural provider who treats the entire community

    b. Specialist physician with long term interaction with patient

    c. Psychiatrist treating patient for years

    d. All of the above

Answer: a. Opinions differ regarding doctors and their former patients. Some argue that such relationships may be permissible for specialists, urgent care providers, or emergency physicians who see a patient once and then terminate ongoing physician patient interaction. While some providers feel that these types of physicians should wait several months before initiating a romantic relationship, others argue that this is not necessary if the medical care relationship has been completed. For rural physicians who are the only health providers in a region, it may be impossible to ban patient relationships altogether. These providers care for the entire local population, so it may be unreasonable to restrict them to long distance relationships.

51. Which of the following is a challenge associated with ethical decision making in health?

    a. Insurance coverage

    b. Rationing of scarce resources

c. Cost control

d. All of the above

Answer: d. As the previous chapters have shown, doctors are faced with ethical choices every day during their practice of medicine, clinical research, or in their educational roles. Their decisions may be time sensitive, sometimes requiring decisions within hours or minutes. Ethical dilemmas vary in their gravity or impact - is it a life or death situation? Will the patient's quality of life be impacted in some way? And they may be juggling cost control issues imposed by their workplace that could influence their prescribing or lead to denial of care based on a patient's insurance coverage or lack thereof for certain treatments and procedures.

52. What is the second step a physician should take for effective decision making when faced with an ethical dilemma?

    a. Recognize that the decision is an ethical dilemma

    b. Gather information

    c. Counsel the patient

    d. Consult an ethics committee

Answer: b. Physicians must first recognize that they face an ethical dilemma and identify the decision to be made. They must then gather information from the patient, consultants, and colleagues. Alternative choices must be identified and weighed against the information pertaining to the case at hand. The physician and patient, or their representative, must then choose from among the choices and take action.

53. Which of the following are accepted rules for ethical conduct for physicians?

    a. The golden rule

    b. The impartiality test

    c. Interpersonal justifiability

    d. All of the above

Answer: d. The golden rule refers to reciprocity as described by the classic phrase, do unto others as you would have done unto you. The impartiality tests means that doctors provide care without any distinction or discrimination, with the added significance of giving priority to those most in need. The universalizability test asks if a provider would feel comfortable if all practitioners acted similarly. The interpersonal justifiability test asks if a physician can provide good reasons for their action that their peers would understand and agree with.

54. Which of the following is a definition of the golden rule test?
    a. Reciprocity
    b. Providing good reasons
    c. Care without prejudice or discrimination
    d. Provider would be comfortable if all physicians acted the same

Answer: a. The golden rule refers to reciprocity as described by the classic phrase, do unto others as you would have done unto you. The impartiality tests means that doctors provide care without any distinction or discrimination, with the added significance of giving priority to those most in need. The universalizability test asks if a provider would feel comfortable if all practitioners acted similarly. The interpersonal justifiability test asks if a physician can provide good reasons for their action that their peers would understand and agree with.

55. Which of the following is a definition of the universalizability test?
    a. Reciprocity
    b. Providing good reasons
    c. Care without prejudice or discrimination
    d. Provider would be comfortable if all physicians acted the same

Answer: d. The golden rule refers to reciprocity as described by the classic phrase, do unto others as you would have done unto you. The impartiality tests means that doctors provide care without any distinction or discrimination, with the added significance of giving priority to those most in need. The universalizability test asks if a provider would feel comfortable if all practitioners acted similarly. The interpersonal justifiability test asks if a physician can provide good reasons for their action that their peers would understand and agree with.

56. When is START triage used?

    a. During busy times

    b. During holiday season

    c. During a mass casualty incident

    d. All of the above

Answer: c. First responders and doctors that are involved in mass-casualty situations deal with ethical dilemmas and are required to make care decisions quickly and efficiently. They do this by using a method called START triage - which stands for simple triage and rapid treatment. Using this method, victims are quickly classified based on the severity of their injuries. This sometimes means that they have to purposefully leave some behind. This triage method was developed in 1983 and is currently widely used across the US. First responders that arrive at a mass-casualty scene quickly assess the victims and classify them into 4 categories that are color-coded as red for immediate care, yellow for delayed care, green for minor care, and black for deceased or beyond treatment. The colors represent triage tags, but actual tags do not have to be used if victims can be physically sorted in different areas. The method is primarily used to determine who gets treated and who gets evacuated to a hospital first. A live patient triaged as black will not be transported and will be allowed to die in the field.

57. What are the consequences of providing futile care?

    a. Higher healthcare costs

    b. Increased pain

    c. Increased suffering

    d. All of the above

Answer: d. At the end of life for patients with terminal conditions, providing certain types of healthcare is considered a futile exercise or of no medical benefit. In some cases, providing healthcare can be considered harmful if associated with pain and complications without any expected benefit. In cases of disagreement with regard to the care provided in end of life decision making, the autonomy principle should guide the care received. While the right to refuse care by patients is often followed without any caveats, when patients demand care in the face of futility it is difficult for health providers to refuse to provide it.

58. What hospital board can evaluate the ethics of research using human subjects?

   a. Institutional review board

   b. Hospital ethics committee

   c. Legal department

   d. Office of the hospital CEO

Answer: a. Institutional review board evaluate and approve research study protocols. These boards are administrative bodies created to protect the rights and welfare of human participants of research studies. They can be established by research institutes, government funding bodies, universities, or individual health facilities. Research studies may need approval from multiple review boards before they can commence. For example, an NIH funded study carried out by a university in a hospital may need separate approval from the NIH, the university, and the hospital in question.

59. Which of the following guide research ethics pertaining to human subjects?

   a. US Food and Drug Administration

   b. National Institutes of Health

   c. European Charter for Researchers

   d. All of the above

Answer: d. Medical research most often refers to interventional research methods, such as clinical trials related to new therapies. Clinical trials are used to evaluate the efficacy of drugs, vaccines, or medical devices for future use by the general public. Because of their invasive nature, clinical trials are heavily regulated by many different agencies, agreements, and laws. Those performing research on human subjects are bound by the principles espoused by these international agreements. These include the Declaration of Helsinki, the Nuremberg Code, national laws and regulations, as well as local requirements by institutional or hospital review boards. In the United States, organizations like the Food and Drug Association and the National Institutes of Health provide oversight over this process. There are also recommended good practice documents, such as the European Charter for Researchers, which provide a framework of best practices when working with human subjects.

60. What is the main issue pertaining to an individual's right to be safe from harmful effects of a study?

    a. Beneficence

    b. Nonmaleficence

    c. Autonomy

    d. Justice

Answer: b. Research involving human subjects is often invasive, requiring individuals to take medications, comply with certain lifestyle changes, and be monitored and probed. Some of these individuals may suffer painful side effects, stress, and other symptoms as a result of the research. For this reason, researchers must consider the costs and benefits of performing the experiment. In other words, the potential benefits of the research must far outweigh the costs to participants. During research studies with human subjects, the intent is not only to try to achieve good by developing a new drug, vaccine or medical device/technique that will eventually improve people's lives, but also to minimize the negative effects of the experiments on participants.

61. Which of the following specific groups were targeted by Nazi Experiments?

    a. Political Dissidents

    b. The Disabled

    c. Jews

    d. All of the above

Answer: d. The Nazi experimentation on human subjects during World War II is perhaps one of the most globally recognized abuses of the principles of informed consent and nonmaleficence. The Nazis performed painful, often sadistic experiments on many people they considered subhuman, including Jewish people, the Roma, homosexuals, disabled individuals, and political dissidents.

62. Where were the trials of Nazi war crimes held?

    a. Nuremberg

    b. London

c. New York

d. Berlin

Answer: a. At the end of the war, a series of military tribunals were held in Nuremberg, Germany charging many in the Nazi leadership with war crimes. The Nuremberg trials began with the indictments of twenty three Nazi physicians involved in genocide and unethical experimentation in concentration camps. These physicians were also charged with sterilizing over three million people to eliminate so-called genetic defects from the German gene pool.

63. Which of the following documents is considered a basis of the Nuremberg Code

   a. The Finland Declaration

   b. The FDA Code of Research Ethics

   c. The Hippocratic Oath

   d. The Vienna Protocol

Answer: c. Shortly after the Nuremberg trials, the judges used six of the arguments developed by the expert medical advisors for the prosecution to lay out what would eventually become the Nuremberg Code on research ethics. The judges included an additional four points, ultimately outlining ten principles to be applied to medical research involving human subjects. With a focus on informed consent, beneficence, and nonmaleficence, these principles are thought to be based on the Hippocratic Oath.

64. Which ethical code was designed in 1964 to govern medical research?

   a. The Berlin Code

   b. The London Protocol

   c. The Helsinki Declaration

   d. The NIH Protocol

Answer: c. Nearly two decades after the Nuremberg Trials, the international community came together to further evaluate the state of ethics related to research. The Declaration of Helsinki is a set of ethics principles developed by the World Medicine Association (WMA) in Helsinki, Finland in 1964. The Declaration of Helsinki represents the first time that the medical community came together to develop standards for human research in an effort self-regulate. Although it does not have binding power in international law, the Declaration of Helsinki is widely considered one of the most influential documents on human research ethics to this day, influencing countless national and regional laws and regulations governing researching ethics. The document has since been revised multiple times, and focuses on an individual's right to self-determination and informed consent, that the participant's well-being takes precedence over the science, and that ethical considerations come before laws and regulations.

65. What disease was studied during the Tuskegee experiments?

    a. HIV

    b. Chlamydia

    c. Gonorrhea

    d. Syphilis

Answer: d. From the 1930s to the 1970s, the United States Public Health Service began studying a group of over six hundred African American men in collaboration with Tuskegee University. A large proportion of the men were already infected with Syphilis, and the study secretly aimed to determine how and when individuals infected with syphilis should be treated. During the experiments, the men were told they were being treated for "bad blood," a colloquialism referring to several different diseases including syphilis and anemia. The researchers notably did not inform the individuals with syphilis of their condition. Furthermore, even after it was known that penicillin was an effective treatment for syphilis, the men were not appropriately treated, and were even prevented from seeking treatment.

66. Why are HeLa cells considered valuable?

    a. Cells divide faster and can be kept alive longer

    b. Cells divide slower and can be kept alive forever

    c. Cells never mutate and can be kept alive longer

    d. Cells never divide and are immune to all antibiotics

Answer: a. In 1951, Henrietta Lacks was biopsied for a cervical cancer tumor at Johns Hopkins Hospital. During the course of her treatment, samples of her cervix were taken without her permission or knowledge. The samples were given to George Otto Gey, a physician and cancer researcher. While he was studying Lacks' tumor, he noticed that her cells divided at a higher rate than most cells and could be kept alive for longer periods of time.

67. How many patents are based on HeLa cells?
    a. One Hundred
    b. One Thousand
    c. More than Ten Thousand
    d. None

Answer: c. HeLa cells are known as "immortal cells," capable of dividing many times and allowing researchers to perform extensive experiments on the same line of cells. This added considerable value to controlled experiments by eliminating the additional variable of experimenting on different cells. They are now one of the most widely used cell lines in medical research and have become commercially successful with over 11,000 patents on her cells. HeLa cells have been used in countless experiments around the world, including research on cancer and HIV, and have helped advance medical science.

68. What type of stem cell can be induced to divide and differentiate into only limited cell types?
    a. Adult Stem Cells
    b. Cardiac Cells
    c. Embryonic Stem Cells
    d. Liver Cells

Answer: a. There are two main types of stem cells: adult and embryonic cells. Following fertilization of an embryo, at the early stages of cell division, stem cells are considered totipotent - able to divide and differentiate into any cell in the body, as well as placental cells. Adult stem cells may be induced to become pluripotent - to differentiate into multiple different cell types in the body.

69. What type of stem cell can be induced to divide and differentiate into only limited cell types?

    a. Totipotent Stem Cells

    b. Pluripotent Stem Cells

    c. Embryonic Stem Cells

    d. Liver Cells

Answer: b. There are two main types of stem cells: adult and embryonic cells. Following fertilization of an embryo, at the early stages of cell division, stem cells are considered totipotent - able to divide and differentiate into any cell in the body, as well as placental cells. Adult stem cells may be induced to become pluripotent - to differentiate into multiple different cell types in the body.

70. What type of stem cell can be induced to divide and differentiate into any cell type?

    a. Totipotent Stem Cells

    b. Pluripotent Stem Cells

    c. Bone Marrow Stem Cells

    d. Liver Cells

Answer: a. There are two main types of stem cells: adult and embryonic cells. Following fertilization of an embryo, at the early stages of cell division, stem cells are considered totipotent - able to divide and differentiate into any cell in the body, as well as placental cells. Adult stem cells may be induced to become pluripotent - to differentiate into multiple different cell types in the body.

71. Which of the following is a definition of ethics?

    a. Legal precedent based on case history

    b. Hospital procedures

    c. The framework to evaluate right versus wrong

    d. All of the above

Answer: c. Ethics can be defined as the framework to evaluate right versus wrong decisions according to an agreed upon set of underlying values. Medical ethics is the application of these principles to the field of clinical care and research.

72. Who was Hippocrates?

    a. A roman emperor

    b. A Greek king

    c. An American President

    d. A Greek physician

Answer: d. Hippocrates was a physician in ancient Greece and is often considered to be the father of the medical profession.

73. When was the original Hippocratic Oath first written?

    a. 10th century BC

    b. 3rd Century BC

    c. 1776

    d. 1964

Answer: b. The original oath that bears his name dates back to the third century BC and has been updated several times to reflect the ages. The modern version most frequently used by medical school graduates was written in 1964.

74. Which of the following is a core principle of medical ethics?

    a. Duty

    b. Honor

    c. Care

    d. Justice

Answer: d. Justice is a core principle of medical ethics.

75. Which of the following is a thought experiment commonly used to teach ethics?

    a. Game Theory

    b. Prisoner's dilemma

    c. Trolley experiment

    d. All of the above

Answer: c. According to the trolley problem, a driver of a trolley or streetcar notices that the brakes have failed. Ahead of him on the track are five people who will be struck and killed if he does nothing. He has the ability to switch to an adjacent track, but that will mean killing a single person who is standing on track number two. So what action should the driver take?

76. Which of the following are "virtues" according to virtue ethics?
    a. Patient Centered Care
    b. Cowardice
    c. Recklessness
    d. Courage

Answer: d. Courage is a virtue according to virtue ethics.

77. Which phrase summarizes the principle of utilitarianism?
    a. The ends justify the means
    b. From each according to their abilities
    c. First do no harm
    d. To each according to their needs

Answer: a. Utilitarianism, also known as consequentialism, evaluates decisions based on their outcomes, or consequences. An ethical action or decision, utilizing this approach, would therefore be the one that does the most good or the least harm in a given situation. Put another way, an ethical action is one that produces a positive outcome.

78. What should a physician do when a child is brought to the ER without a caregiver if the child is in stable condition?
    a. Wait for a legal guardian to authorize any treatment
    b. Administer care and then contact a parent
    c. Administer care while attempting to contact a parent
    d. Do not contact their parent

Answer: a. As a general rule, a physician must obtain parental consent for minors, meaning any patient under the age of eighteen. The need for consent can be waived in the case of a life threatening or potentially life threatening condition. So, for example, epinephrine for a child presenting to the emergency room with an anaphylactic reaction should not be withheld while awaiting a call back from the child's parents. Conversely, a child with a stable medical complaint brought to the emergency room from school should not be treated until permission is obtained from their legal guardian.

79. Which NFL star caused a scandal when he presented to the ER with a gunshot wound and the ER did not make a timely report to the police?
    a. Joe Namath
    b. Plaxico Burress
    c. Joe Montana
    d. John Riggins

Answer: b. Physicians and hospitals can be severely penalized for not reporting certain cases when legally required to do so. In 2008, an NFL star athlete named Plaxico Burress accidentally shot himself with an unlicensed firearm. He contacted a local hospital in New York City before his arrival to seek care. The hospital then proceeded to knowingly provide him with treatment under an assumed name. The hospital and treating physician subsequently failed to notify law enforcement for nearly eight hours, and by that time the patient had already been discharged.

80. What should a physician do if they suspect child abuse in a patient?
    a. Confront the parent
    b. Perform an investigation
    c. Report the case to authorities
    d. Maintain confidentiality

Answer: c. Cases of child abuse are an example where confidentiality must be breached. Medical decision making for children is, under normal circumstances, the responsibility of their adult legal guardians. In a circumstance where a medical provider suspects abuse, or

171

when the child reports abuse to the provider, the provider is obligated to report the case to the police or other child welfare authority.

81. Which of the following may be a case that must be reported to authorities depending on local law?
    a. Child abuse
    b. Elder abuse
    c. Impaired driver
    d. All of the above

Answer. D. All of the above may require reporting to authorities.

82. Which of the following scenarios are suspicious for child abuse and should be reported to child welfare authorities?
    a. Retinal hemorrhages
    b. Spiral forearm fracture in 2 year old who fell from bed
    c. Multiple old healing injuries
    d. All of the above

Answer: d. Cases of child abuse are another example where confidentiality must be breached. In a circumstance where a medical provider suspects abuse, or when the child reports abuse to the provider, the provider is obligated to report the case to the police or other child welfare authority. This scenario often arises with the injuries of a child do not match the history of the event provided by the child or family member. Concerning findings on physical examination may also arouse suspicion, including spiral bone fractures, retinal hemorrhages, and multiple old injuries at various stages of healing.

83. Which of the following is considered protected health information or PHI?
    a. Photograph
    b. Digital x-ray images
    c. Diagnosis billing code
    d. Laboratory result

Answer: a. PHI includes any information that can be used to link a medical record to an individual. While the medical record includes health conditions and treatments, patient identifiers under this framework include a patient's name, date of birth, social security number, medical record number, address, email, and photograph.

84. What medical technology increases the risk of sex selection and skewed male female ratios?
    a. Amniocentesis
    b. Ultrasound
    c. X-Ray
    d. CT Scan

Answer: b. Ultrasound can be used to identify the sex of the fetus.

85. Which of the following are types of sterilization?
    a. Vasectomy
    b. In-Vitro Fertilization
    c. Sperm Donation
    d. All of the above

Answer: a. A vasectomy is a surgical procedure for men. It consists of cutting the vas deferens – which are the tubes that carry sperm from the testicles to the prostate. This prevents the sperm from entering semen, hence rendering a man unable to reproduce since their ejaculate will be devoid of sperm.

86. How is euthanasia different from physician assisted suicide?
    a. In Euthanasia a doctor refused to harm a patient
    b. In Physician Assisted Suicide a doctor administers medications
    c. In Euthanasia a doctor administers medications
    d. All of the above

Answer: c. In Euthanasia a doctor does more than provide a prescription, they actually administer the medications.

87. What should a doctor do in case of a medical error?

    a. Hide all evidence

    b. Report the error to the police

    c. Call their lawyer

    d. Admit to the error and apologize

Answer: d. According to prevailing ethical standards and the need to preserve trust in the doctor patient relationship, all medical errors should be disclosed to patients immediately. Numerous studies have demonstrated that immediate disclosure along with an apology results in fewer malpractice lawsuits related to errors.

88. Which of the following is a conflict of interest?

    a. Physician owns stock in a company whose products they promotes to their patients

    b. Physician cares for their family members

    c. Physician orders tests and directs patients to their relative's laboratory

    d. All of the above

Answer: d. All of the above are potential conflicts of interest.

89. When does the doctor patient relationship begin?

    a. When a patient is referred to a doctor

    b. When a patient makes an appointment to see a doctor

    c. When a doctor provides treatment recommendations via a telephone consultation while on call

    d. All of the above

Answer: c. Physicians who have begun treatment, performed an examination, made a recommendation, or made a verbal agreement to take action as a doctor on call or consultant physician however, have in fact begun a care relationship so are obligated to continue care according their responsibility as the treating physician.

90. What type of doctor cannot refuse to treat a patient requesting their care while on duty?

a. Neurologist

b. Pediatrician

c. Emergency Physician

d. Obstetrician

Answer: c. The right to refuse care does not apply to doctors working in an emergency room, who must treat all potential patients. It is also not permitted to refuse treatment based on a personal characteristic of the patient as that would be defined as discrimination.

91. What is a common cause of physician impairment?

a. Alcohol abuse

b. Conflict of interest

c. Financial hardship

d. Family member illness

Answer: a. Physicians as a group suffer from the same challenges faced by the general population including alcohol and drug abuse, psychiatric illness, and dementia. Alcohol abuse is the most common cause of physician impairment. An estimated eight to twelve percent of physicians will suffer from some form of substance abuse during the course of their careers. Physicians working in the specialties of emergency medicine and anesthesiology are considered to have the highest risk of substance abuse compared with others. Impaired physicians place their patients at risk of medical errors and inappropriate care every day they continue to practice.

92. If a physician suspects a colleague is impaired, who can they make a report to?

a. The doctor's patients

b. The police

c. State licensing board

d. The doctor's spouse

Answer: c. Physicians have an obligation to report colleagues they believe may be impaired to the appropriate authorities, including their department administration, hospital management, and state licensing board. Many states have license immunity programs where physicians who voluntary seek care for substance abuse are protected from losing their license if they follow a defined counseling and rehabilitation program.

93. Which of the following gifts may be acceptable for a doctor to accept?
    a. Baked goods during the holidays
    b. A Rolex watch
    c. A new car
    d. All of the above

Answer: a. Most physicians choose the conditional acceptance of gifts. When evaluating an individual gift, they can consider the motivation of the patient in giving it. Is the patient trying to secure preferential treatment? Is the gift itself an inappropriate item indicating romance or other intimacy? Is the gift extravagant? Physicians can also consider the timing of the gift. A gift given in late December for example, may be appropriate and in line with cultural norms of seasonal gift giving.

94. What is the term for physicians moving from poor countries to rich countries?
    a. Brain drain
    b. Brain circulation
    c. Brain freeze
    d. Brain attack

Answer: a. Many developing countries are suffering from the brain drain, which is defined as a migration of highly skilled health professionals from low income to high income countries.

95. What is the term for rich countries benefiting from the health workers trained in poor countries?
    a. Brain freeze
    b. Brain circulation
    c. Brain gain
    d. Brain attack

Answer: c. Many developing countries are suffering from the brain drain, which is defined as a migration of highly skilled health professionals from low income to high income countries. On the receiving end are the high-income countries who reap a brain gain from immigration of these highly skilled professionals.

96. Approximately how much is spent on medicines in the United States?
    a. $10 million
    b. $125 million
    c. $150 billion
    d. $450 billion

Answer: d. In the United States alone, we spend around $450 billion on medicines. The pharmaceutical industry is growing at a fast rate, but many criticize their pricing policies and availability of drugs.

97. When was polio eradicated?
    a. 1901
    b. 1964
    c. 2010
    d. Polio has not been eradicated

Answer: d. Polio has not yet been eradicated and as of 2018 remains active in the wild-type form in Afghanistan and Pakistan.

98. Which of the following is not a form of sterilization?
    a. Tubal ligation
    b. In-Vitro Fertilization
    c. Vasectomy
    d. Hysterectomy and oophorectomy

Answer: b. IVF is a way to induce pregnancy, not sterilize individuals.

99. Which of the following is a core principle of medical ethics?
    a. Academics

b. Clinical Care

c. Honesty

d. Beneficence

Answer: d. Beneficence is a core principle of medical ethics.

100.   When was the modern Hippocratic Oath written?

a. 10th century BC

b. 3rd Century BC

c. 1776

d. 1964

Answer: d. The original oath that bears his name dates back to the third century BC and has been updated several times to reflect the ages. The modern version most frequently used by medical school graduates was written in 1964.

Made in the USA
Monee, IL
30 August 2022